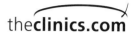

CLINICS IN LIVER DISEASE

Alcoholic Liver Disease

GUEST EDITOR
Carroll B. Leevy, MD

CONSULTING EDITOR
Norman Gitlin, MD

February 2005 • Volume 9 • Number 1

SAUNDERS

An Imprint of Elsevier, Inc.
PHILADELPHIA   LONDON   TORONTO   MONTREAL   SYDNEY   TOKYO

W.B. SAUNDERS COMPANY
A Division of Elsevier Inc.

The Curtis Center • Independence Square West • Philadelphia, Pennsylvania 19106

http://www.theclinics.com

CLINICS IN LIVER DISEASE　　　　　　　　　　Volume 9, Number 1
February 2005　　　　　　　　　　　　　　　　　　ISSN 1089-3261
Editor: Kerry Holland　　　　　　　　　　　　　ISBN 1-4160-2778-5

1 00502053 5

The ideas and opinions expressed in *Clinics in Liver Disease* do not necessarily reflect those of the Publisher. The Publisher does not assume any responsibility for any injury and/or damage to persons or property arising out of or related to any use of the material contained in this periodical. The reader is advised to check the appropriate medical literature and the product information currently provided by the manufacturer of each drug to be administered to verify the dosage, the method and duration of administration, or contraindications. It is the responsibility of the treating physician or other health care professional, relying on independent experience and knowledge of the patient, to determine drug dosages and the best treatment for the patient. Mention of any product in this issue should not be construed as endorsement by the contributors, editors, or the Publisher of the product or manufacturers' claims.

Clinics in Liver Disease (ISSN 1089-3261) is published quarterly by W.B. Saunders Company. Corporate and editorial offices: The Curtis Center, Independence Square West, Philadelphia, PA 19106-3399. Accounting and circulation offices: 6277 Sea Harbor Drive, Orlando, FL 32887-4800. Periodicals pending postage paid at Orlando, FL 32862, and additional mailing offices. Subscription prices are $165.00 per year (U.S. individuals), $83.00 per year (U.S. student/resident), $234.00 per year (U.S. institutions), $205.00 per year (foreign individuals), $103.00 per year (foreign student/resident), $273.00 per year (foreign institutions), $188.00 per year (Canadian individuals), and $273.00 per year (Canadian institutions). Foreign air speed delivery is included in all *Clinics* subscription prices. All prices are subject to change without notice. POSTMASTER: Send address changes to *Clinics in Liver Disease*, W.B. Saunders Company, Periodicals Fulfillment, Orlando, FL 32887-4800. **Customer Service: 1-800-654-2452** (US). From outside of the US, call **407-345-4000**. E-mail: hhspcs@harcourt.com.

Reprints. For copies of 100 or more, of articles in this publication, please contact the Commercial Reprints Department, Elsevier Inc., 360 Park Avenue South, New York, New York 10010-1710. Tel. (212) 633-3813 Fax: (212) 462-1935 e-mail: reprints@elsevier.com.

Clinics in Liver Disease is covered in *Index Medicus*.

Printed in the United States of America

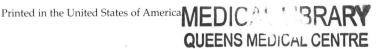

CONSULTING EDITOR

NORMAN GITLIN, MD, Professor of Medicine, Atlanta Gastroenterology Associates, Crawford Long Hospital: An Emory Affiliate, Atlanta, Georgia

GUEST EDITOR

CARROLL B. LEEVY, MD, Professor and Scientific Director, University of Medicine and Dentistry of New Jersey–Newark, New Jersey Medical School, Liver Center, Sammy Davis Jr. National Liver Institute, Newark, New Jersey

CONTRIBUTORS

SRIPRIYA BALASUBRAMANIAN, MD, Division of Gastroenterology and Hepatology, University of California at Davis, Sacramento, California

HANY A. ELBESHBESHY, MD, University of Medicine and Dentistry of New Jersey–Newark, New Jersey Medical School, Liver Center, Sammy Davis Jr. National Liver Institute, Newark, New Jersey

CARROLL B. LEEVY, MD, Professor and Scientific Director, University of Medicine and Dentistry of New Jersey–Newark, New Jersey Medical School, Liver Center, Sammy Davis Jr. National Liver Institute, Newark, New Jersey

CARROLL M. LEEVY, MD, University of Medicine and Dentistry of New Jersey Distinguished Professor and Scientific Director, Sammy Davis Jr. National Liver Institute, New Jersey Medical School Liver Center, University of Medicine and Dentistry, Newark, New Jersey

JAY H. LEFKOWITCH, MD, Professor of Clinical Pathology, Department of Surgical Pathology, College of Physicians and Surgeons, Columbia University, New York, New York

CHARLES S. LIEBER, MD, MACP, Professor, Departments of Medicine and Pathology, Mount Sinai School of Medicine; and Chief, Section of Liver Disease and Nutrition, Alcohol Research and Treatment Center, Bronx VA Medical Center, Bronx, New York

KRIS V. KOWDLEY, MD, Division of Gastroenterology and Hepatology, University of Washington, Seattle, Washington

ARTHUR J. McCULLOUGH, MD, Director, Division of Gastroenterology, MetroHealth Medical Center; and Professor of Medicine, Case Western Reserve University, Cleveland, Ohio

ŞERBAN A. MOROIANU, MD, Sammy Davis Jr. National Liver Institute, New Jersey Medical School Liver Center, University of Medicine and Dentistry, Newark, New Jersey

KEVIN D. MULLEN, MD, Professor of Medicine, Case Western Reserve School of Medicine, Cleveland, Ohio

ROBERT S. O'SHEA, MD, MSCE, Assistant Professor of Medicine, Cleveland Clinic, Lerner College of Medicine, Cleveland, Ohio

MICHAEL D. VOIGT, MBCHB, M MED, FCP(SA), Medical Director, Liver Failure and Transplantation, University of Iowa Hospitals and Clinics, Iowa City; and Professor of Medicine, Department of Medicine, Lucille A. and Roy J. Carver College of Medicine, Iowa City, Iowa

JAMILÉ WAKIM-FLEMING, MD, Assistant Professor, Case Western Reserve School of Medicine, Cleveland, Ohio

ROWEN K. ZETTERMAN, MD, MACP, FACG, Chief of Staff, Nebraska-Western Iowa VA Health Care Center, Omaha; and The University of Nebraska Medical Center–Omaha, Omaha, Nebraska

CONTRIBUTORS

CONTENTS

Preface   xi
Carroll B. Leevy

Metabolism of Alcohol   1
Charles S. Lieber

Most tissues of the body contain enzymes capable of ethanol oxidation or nonoxidative metabolism, but significant activity occurs only in the liver and, to a lesser extent, in the stomach. Hence, medical consequences are predominant in these organs. In the liver, ethanol oxidation generates an excess of reducing equivalents, primarily as NADH, causing hepatotoxicity. An additional system, containing cytochromes P-450 inducible by chronic alcohol feeding, was demonstrated in liver microsomes and found to be a major cause of hepatotoxicity.

Morphology of Alcoholic Liver Disease   37
Jay H. Lefkowitch

The major pathologic manifestations of alcoholic liver injury have been well described and include three major lesions: steatosis (fatty liver), steatohepatitis (formerly alcoholic hepatitis), and cirrhosis. Recent attention to the problem of nonalcoholic fatty liver disease (NAFLD) in individuals with obesity, diabetes, and other risk factors has shed light on the mechanisms of cellular injury associated with hepatic steatosis and on the potential pathways to steatohepatitis and cirrhosis. Pathologists need to be familiar with the spectrum of changes seen in steatohepatitis, including hepatocyte ballooning, Mallory bodies, mixed inflammatory cell infiltrates, and a distinctive perivenular and pericellular "chicken-wire" fibrosis. These features and other less common histopathologic lesions in the liver are reviewed and illustrated.

Immunology of Alcoholic Liver Disease 55
Carroll B. Leevy and Hany A. Elbeshbeshy

Alcohol-induced liver injury is a reflection of the immunologic response of the liver to this stimulus. Reported studies of immunologic abnormalities in alcoholic liver disease (ALD) patients suggest that immunologic response plays a key role in the pathogenesis of chronic liver disease in alcoholics, and have contributed to the understanding of how some patients with ALD progress into alcoholic liver cirrhosis. The immunologic response of the liver is reflected in alcoholic fatty liver disease, hyaline necrosis, and cirrhosis, promoted by the role of neutrophils in damaging liver cells through cytotoxicity, and lymphocytes through cytotoxicity, inducing fibrogenesis of the liver and formation of immune complexes responsible for immune complex-mediated cytotoxicity, in addition to the role of different chemokines in attracting leucocytes, inducing fibrogenesis and liver cell apoptosis, with the established mechanism by which Mallory bodies evoke both cellular and humoral immunity contributing to the process of alcoholic liver cirrhosis, which plays a key role in transformation of alcoholic hepatitis to cirrhosis. At present, research is underway to find modalities to correct the induced immunologic changes, so at this time, it is necessary to avoid alcoholism, with the use of social and educational programs to stop alcoholism.

Nutritional Aspects of Alcoholic Liver Disease 67
Carroll M. Leevy and Şerban A. Moroianu

Development of ethanol-induced fatty liver, alcoholic hepatitis, and cirrhosis has been attributed in part to nutritional deficiencies for many years. Special attention must be focused on treating alcohol-induced liver disease while providing replacement of deficient amino acids, vitamins, minerals, and other nutrients. Avoidance of alcohol intake is required to eliminate progressive liver disease in alcoholics. This is best achieved by using educational and social programs to convince patients and their caretakers of the great necessity to eliminate alcohol intake.

Effect of Alcohol on Viral Hepatitis and Other Forms of Liver Dysfunction 83
Sripriya Balasubramanian and Kris V. Kowdley

Alcohol is a known hepatotoxic agent, which may exacerbate liver injury caused by other agents. The wide prevalence of alcohol use and abuse in society makes it an important cofactor in many other liver diseases. Examples of liver diseases that are significantly influenced by ingestion of alcohol include chronic viral hepatitis, disorders of iron overload, and obesity-related liver disease.

Treatment of Alcoholic Hepatitis 103
Robert S. O'Shea and Arthur J. McCullough

Cirrhosis and its sequelae are responsible for close to 2% of all causes of death in the United States. Some studies have suggested that the costs of liver disease may account for as much as 1% of all health care spending, with alcohol-related liver disease (ALD) representing a major portion. It accounts for between 40% to 50% of all deaths due to cirrhosis, with an accompanying rate of progression of up to 60% in patients with pure alcoholic fatty liver over 10 years, and a 5-year survival rate as low as 35% if patients continue to drink. A subset of patients with ALD will develop an acute, virulent form of injury, acute alcoholic hepatitis, which has a substantially worse prognosis. Despite enormous progress in understanding the physiology of this disease, much remains unknown, and therefore, a consensus regarding effective therapy for ALD is lacking. Conventional therapy is still based largely on abstinence from alcohol, as well as general supportive and symptomatic care. Unfortunately, hepatocellular damage may progress despite these measures. Multiple treatment interventions for both the short- and long-term morbidity and mortality of this disease have been proposed, but strong disagreement exists among experts regarding the value of any of the proposed specific therapeutic interventions.

Long-Term Management of Alcoholic Liver Disease 135
Jamilé Wakim-Fleming and Kevin D. Mullen

Despite the epidemics of viral hepatitis C and nonalcoholic fatty liver, alcohol remains one of the major causes of liver disease. Commonly, hepatitis C and other liver diseases are found in association with alcohol consumption. This association in many instances is noted to accelerate the progression of liver disease. In many respects, the long-term management of alcoholic liver disease is not dissimilar from the long-term management of patients with cirrhosis from other etiologies. One major element is the abstinence of alcohol use. The ability to maintain sobriety has a major impact on the outcome of patients with alcoholic cirrhosis because maintaining abstinence can lead to significant regression of fibrosis and possibly early cirrhosis. Similarities in managing patients with cirrhosis due to alcohol or cirrhosis from other causes include vaccination to prevent superimposed viral hepatitis and screening for esophageal varices and hepatocellular carcinoma with subsequent appropriate therapy.

Alcohol in Hepatocellular Cancer 151
Michael D. Voigt

Hepatocellular cancer accounts for almost half a million cancer deaths a year, with an escalating incidence in the Western world. Alcohol has long been recognized as a major risk factor for cancer of the liver and of other organs including oropharynx, larynx, esophagus, and possibly the breast and colon. There is compelling epidemiologic data confirming the increased risk of cancer associated with alcohol consumption, which is supported by animal experiments. Cancer of the liver associated with alcohol usually occurs in the setting of cirrhosis. Alcohol may act as a cocarcinogen, and has strong synergistic effects with other carcinogens including hepatitis B and C, aflatoxin, vinyl chloride, obesity, and diabetes mellitus. Acetaldehyde, the main metabolite of alcohol, causes hepatocellular injury, and is an important factor in causing increased oxidant stress, which damages DNA. Alcohol affects nutrition and vitamin metabolism, causing abnormalities of DNA methylation. Abnormalities of DNA methylation, a key pathway of epigenetic gene control, lead to cancer. Other nutritional and metabolic effects, for example on vitamin A metabolism, also play a key role in hepatocarcinogenesis. Alcohol enhances the effects of environmental carcinogens directly and by contributing to nutritional deficiency and impairing immunologic tumor surveillance. This review summarizes the epidemiologic evidence for the role of alcohol in hepatocellular cancer, and discusses the mechanisms involved in the promotion of cancer.

Liver Transplantation for Alcoholic Liver Disease 171
Rowen K. Zetterman

Patients with end-stage alcoholic liver disease should be considered for liver transplantation. A careful pretransplant evaluation must be undertaken to assess for both medical and psychiatric factors that will continue to require attention following transplantation. Although most programs require at least 6 months of ethanol abstinence before consideration of liver transplantation, there is little evidence that this conclusively predicts a reduction in recidivism. Most programs continue to exclude those with alcoholic hepatitis. Postoperatively, attention to psychiatric issues, recidivism, compliance, and assessment for tumors, especially squamous cell carcinomas, should be undertaken.

Index 183

FORTHCOMING ISSUES

May 2005
Hepatocellular Carcinoma
Morris Sherman, MB BCh, PhD, FRCP(C), *Guest Editor*

August 2005
Hepatitis C Virus
Emmet B. Keeffe, MD, *Guest Editor*

November 2005
Recent Advances in the Treatment of Liver Disorders
Jorge Herrera, MD, *Guest Editor*

RECENT ISSUES

November 2004
Metabolic Liver Diseases
Bruce R. Bacon, MD, *Guest Editor*

August 2004
Nonalcoholic Fatty Liver Disease
Arun J. Sanyal, MBBS, MD, *Guest Editor*

May 2004
Hepatitis B
Tram T. Tran, MD, and
Paul Martin, MD, *Guest Editors*

ELSEVIER
SAUNDERS

CLINICS IN
LIVER DISEASE

Clin Liver Dis 9 (2005) xi–xii

Preface

Alcoholic Liver Disease

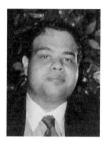

Carroll B. Leevy, MD
Guest Editor

This issue of the *Clinics in Liver Disease* provides an update on the prevention, recognition, and treatment of alcoholic liver disease—a continuing cause of disability and death throughout the world. Alcoholism is a direct cause of fatty liver, hepatitis, cirrhosis and liver cancer; it contributes to the development of hepatitis B and C and the uncovering of congenital hepatic disorders; and it predisposes individuals to toxic liver injury. The contributions to this issue provide an update on the mechanisms of alcohol-induced liver injury, criteria for diagnosis, medical therapy, and transplantation. Knowledge of the contributions of nutrient deficiency and immunologic events are reviewed, as are the treatment of specific clinical biochemical and morphologic features and the use of transplantation for end-stage disease. The ability to eliminate liver failure by replacing a diseased liver with a postmortem normal organ or a lobe of a normal liver represents a miraculous health-restoring event. The problem is the cost and the decision of who is eligible for receipt of a new liver. The International Hepatology Informatics Group recommended use of a computerized expert system [1] that has been developed to facilitate selection of a recipient for a new liver. With alcoholic liver disease this is particularly helpful, but the problem of clinical symptomatology, affordability, and posttransplant avoidance of alcoholism remains an important consideration with end-stage alcoholic liver disease.

1089-3261/05/$ – see front matter © 2005 Elsevier Inc. All rights reserved.
doi:10.1016/j.cld.2004.12.001

At this time, a new approach to alcoholic liver disease is being provided by current research on the abnormalities of liver regeneration. Structural and functional changes observed in experimental animals are now being applied to humans; this has great potential in alcoholic liver disease. This is facilitated by simultaneous perfusion of flash-frozen percutaneous biopsies or explanted liver in any acrylic chamber with tritiated thymidine and proline to evaluate DNA and collagen synthesis, respectively. These investigations indicate that chronic liver damage is associated with replication of mesenchymal, ductular, and parenchymal cells accompanied by increased fibrogenesis [2,3]. The regenerative response of the liver after noxious injury from alcohol is accompanied by cytokines, increased growth response genes, and changes in telomerase activity. The ability to monitor these parameters provides new information on the kinetics of the reparative process and the ability to modify it. Noteworthy is the ability to obtain an index to these changes by studies of subcellular changes in both liver and other tissues from persons who suffer from alcoholism. Therapeutic manipulations of liver regeneration is of key importance. Investigations must be continued to develop more effective measures to detect and modify deficient or excess regeneration after liver injury by alcohol or other agents.

Carroll B. Leevy, MD
University of Medicine and Dentistry of New Jersey
150 Bergen Street, Room H-245
Newark, NJ 07103, USA
E-mail address: leevycb@umdnj.edu

References

[1] Leevy CM, Sherlock S, Tygstrup N, et al. Disease of the liver and biliary tract, standardization of nomenclature, diagnostic criteria and prognosis. New York: Raven Press; 1984.

[2] Leevy CM, NcNeal G, Habba S. Process and apparatus for evaluating liver disease. US Patent No. 4,675,284, 1984.

[3] Leevy CB. Abnormalities of liver regeneration: a review. Dig Dis 1998;16:88–98.

ELSEVIER
SAUNDERS

CLINICS IN
LIVER DISEASE

Clin Liver Dis 9 (2005) 1–35

Metabolism of Alcohol

Charles S. Lieber, MD, MACP

Bronx VA Medical Center (151-2), 130 West Kingsbridge Road, Bronx, NY 10468, USA

Many of the metabolic and toxic effects of alcohol in the liver have been linked to its metabolism in that organ (Fig. 1). Ethanol is readily absorbed from the gastrointestinal tract. Only 2% to 10% of that absorbed is eliminated through the kidneys and lungs; the rest is oxidized in the body, principally in the liver. Except for the stomach, extrahepatic metabolism of ethanol is small. This relative organ specificity, coupled with the high energy content of ethanol (each gram provides 29 kJ, or 7.1 kcal) and the lack of effective feedback control of its rate of hepatic metabolism, may result in a displacement, by ethanol, of up to 90% of the liver's normal metabolic substrates, and probably explains why ethanol disposal produces striking metabolic imbalances in the liver. The extent to which ethanol becomes the preferred fuel for the total body has been demonstrated in humans: it decreased total body fat oxidation by 79% and protein oxidation by 39%, and almost completely abolished the 249% rise in carbohydrate oxidation seen after glucose infusion [1].

Through each of its pathways, ethanol produces specific metabolic and toxic disturbances, and all three pathways result in the production of acetaldehyde, a highly toxic metabolite.

The alcohol dehydrogenase pathway and associated metabolic disorders

ADH isozymes

The major pathway for ethanol disposition involves alcohol dehydrogenase (ADH), an enzyme that catalyzes the conversion of ethanol to acetaldehyde. The *raison d'être* of this enzyme might be to rid the body of the small amounts

Portions of this article appeared previously in Lieber C. Metabolism of alcohol. Clinics in Liver Disease 1998;2(4):673–702; with permission.
E-mail address: liebercs@aol.com

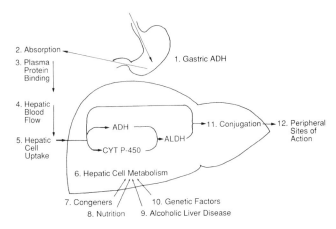

Fig. 1. Schematic illustration of the main pathways of ethanol disposition in stomach and liver. Metabolic and drug interactions may affect conjugation, microsomal cytochrome P-450-dependent pathways (CYT P-450), ADH, and acetaldehyde dehydrogenase (ALDH) (*From* Lieber CS. G.I. pharmacology and therapeutics: alcoholic liver disease. In: Friedman G, Jacobson ED, McCallum RW, editors. Gastrointestinal pharmacology and therapeutics. Philadelphia (PA): Lippincott-Raven Press; 1997. Chapter 35. p. 465–87; with permission.)

of alcohol produced by fermentation in the gut [2]. ADH has a broad substrate specificity, which includes dehydrogenation of steroids, oxidation of the intermediary alcohols of the shunt pathway of mevalonate metabolism, and ω-oxidation of fatty acids [3]; these processes may act as the "physiologic" substrates for ADH.

Human liver ADH is a zinc metalloenzyme with five classes of multiple molecular forms that arise from the association of eight different types of subunits, α, $\beta 1$, $\beta 2$, $\beta 3$, $\gamma 1$, $\gamma 2$, π, and χ, into active dimeric molecules. A genetic model accounts for this multiplicity as products of five gene loci, ADH1 through ADH5 [4]. There are three types of subunit, α, β, and γ in class I. Polymorphism occurs at two loci, ADH2 and ADH3, which encode the β and γ subunits. Class II isozymes migrate more anodically than class I isozymes (Fig. 2) and, unlike the latter, which generally have low K_m values for ethanol, class II (or π) ADH has a relatively high K_m (34 mM) and a relative insensitivity to 4-methylpyrazole inhibition. Class III (χADH) does not participate in the oxidation of ethanol in the liver because of its very low affinity for that substrate; it is not inhibited by 12 mM 4-methylpyrazole [5]. More recently, a new isoenzyme of ADH has been purified from human stomach (vide infra), the so-called σ- or μ-ADH (class IV) [6,7] and a cDNA encoding yet another new form of ADH (class V) in liver and stomach was reported [8].

Metabolic effects of excessive alcohol dehydrogenase-mediated hepatic NADH generation

In ADH-mediated oxidation of ethanol, acetaldehyde is produced and hydrogen is transferred from ethanol to the cofactor nicotinamide adenine di-

COMPARISON OF GASTRIC AND LIVER ADH

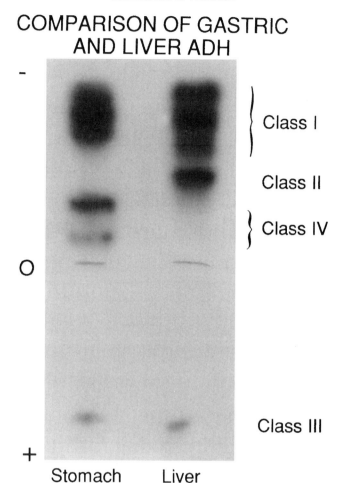

Fig. 2. ADH isoenzymes in cytosol from liver and gastric mucosa obtained during surgery. Class II ADH is present in the liver but not in the stomach. By contrast, two bands of activity with slow cathodic mobility on starch gel electrophoresis are present in the gastric mucosa, but not in the liver. They correspond to class IV, or what has also been called μ- or σ-ADH (*From* Hernández-Muñoz R, Caballeria J, Baraona E, Uppal R, Greenstein R, Lieber CS. Human gastric alcohol dehydrogenase: Its inhibition by H₂-receptor antagonists, and its effect on the bioavailability of ethanol. Alcohol Clin Exp Res 1990;14:946–50.)

nucleotide (NAD), which is converted to its reduced form (NADH) (Fig. 3). The formed acetaldehyde again loses hydrogen and is metabolized to acetate, most of which is released into the bloodstream. As a net result, ethanol oxidation generates an excess of reducing equivalents in the liver, primarily as NADH, and it was postulated that the latter may be involved in the hepatotoxicity [9]. This was corroborated by the observation that the ethanol-induced stimulation of

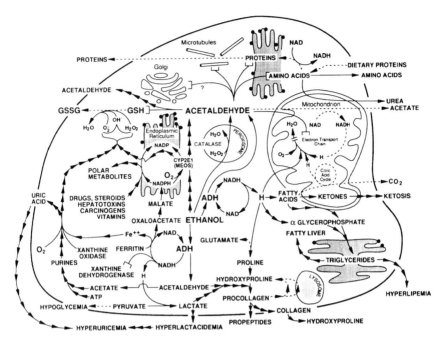

Fig. 3. Oxidation of ethanol in the hepatocyte. Many disturbances in intermediary metabolism and toxic effects can be linked to (1) ADH-mediated generation of NADH, (2) the induction of the activity of microsomal enzymes, especially the MEOS containing cytochrome P-4502E1 (CYP2E1), and (3) acetaldehyde, the product of ethanol oxidation. GSH, reduced glutathione; GSSG oxidized glutathione.—, pathways that are depressed by ethanol; →→stimulation or activation, interference or binding (*From* Hernández-Muñoz R, Caballeria J, Baraona E, Uppal R, Greenstein R, Lieber CS. Human gastric alcohol dehydrogenase: Its inhibition by H_2-receptor antagonists, and its effect on the bioavailability of ethanol. Alcohol Clin Exp Res 1990;14:946–50; with permission.)

lipogenesis and decrease in fatty acid oxidation was prevented by a hydrogen acceptor such as methylene blue, and mimicked by another NADH generating system, such as sorbitol [9,10]. The increased NADH/NAD ratio also raises the concentration of α-glycerophosphate, which favors hepatic triglyceride accumulation by trapping fatty acids. In addition, excess NADH may promote fatty acid synthesis. Theoretically, enhanced lipogenesis can be considered a means for disposing of the excess hydrogen. Some hydrogen equivalents are transferred into mitochondria by various "shuttle" mechanisms. The activity of the citric acid cycle is depressed, partly because of a slowing of the reactions of the cycle that depend on the NAD/NADH ratio, and the mitochondria will use the hydrogen equivalents originating from ethanol, rather than those derived from the oxidation of fatty acids that normally serve as the main energy source of the liver. In their aggregate, these changes favor hepatic fat accumulation (vide infra).

A number of other hepatic and metabolic effects of ethanol can be attributed to the redox change upon the oxidation of ethanol (Fig. 3) [11], including hyperlactacidemia, which contributes to the acidosis and also reduces the capacity of the kidneys to excrete uric acid, leading to secondary hyperuricemia. Alcohol-induced ketosis and acetate-mediated enhanced adenosine triphosphate (ATP) breakdown and purine generation [12] may also promote the hyperuricemia. Hyperuricemia may be related to the common clinical observation that excessive consumption of alcoholic beverages frequently aggravates or precipitates gouty attacks.

Short-term alcohol intoxication occasionally causes severe hypoglycemia, which can result in sudden death. As reviewed elsewhere [11], hypoglycemia is due, in part, to the block of hepatic gluconeogenesis by ethanol, again as a consequence of the increased NADH/NAD ratio in subjects whose glycogen stores are already depleted by starvation or who have preexisting abnormalities in carbohydrate metabolism. However, depending on the conditions, ethanol may accelerate rather than inhibit gluconeogenesis. Indeed, hyperglycemia may also occur in association with alcoholism. Its mechanism is still obscure, but glucose intolerance may be due, at least in part, to decreased peripheral glucose use.

Hepatic steatosis and other zonal effects in the liver

One of the earliest pathologic manifestation of alcohol abuse is the development of a fatty liver. Fatty acids of different origins can accumulate as triglycerides in the liver because of different metabolic disturbances: decreased hepatic release of lipoproteins, increased mobilization of peripheral fat, enhanced hepatic uptake of circulating lipids, enhanced hepatic lipogenesis (vide supra) and, most importantly, decreased fatty acid oxidation, whether as a function of the reduced citric acid cycle activity secondary to the altered redox potential (vide supra) or as a consequence of permanent changes in mitochondrial structure and functions [11,13,14], now documented by breath analysis in alcoholics [15]. In cultured hepatocytes, the increased intracellular accumulation of triacylglycerol in the presence of ethanol was quantitatively accounted for by increased fatty acid uptake, decreased fatty acid oxidation in the tricarboxylic acid cycle, and decreased lipoprotein secretion [16].

A characteristic feature of liver injury in the alcoholic is the predominance of steatosis and other lesions in the perivenular zone, also called centrilobular or zone 3 of the hepatic acinus. The mechanism for this zonal selectivity of the toxic effects involves several distinct and not mutually exclusive mechanisms. The hypoxia hypothesis originated from the observation that liver slices from rats fed alcohol chronically consume more oxygen than those of controls. It was then postulated that the enhanced consumption of oxygen would increase the gradient of oxygen tension along the sinusoids to the extent of producing anoxic injury of perivenular hepatocytes [17]. Indeed, both in human alcoholics [18] and in animals fed alcohol chronically [19,20], decreases in either hepatic venous oxygen saturation [18] or PO_2 [19] and in tissue oxygen tension [20] have been found during the withdrawal state. However, the changes in hepatic oxygenation found during the withdrawal state disappeared [19,21] or decreased [20] when alcohol was present in the blood. Acute ethanol administration increased splanchnic oxygen consumption in naive baboons, but the consequences of this effect on oxygenation in the perivenular zone were offset by increased blood flow, resulting in unchanged hepatic venous oxygen tension [19]. In fact, ethanol induces an increase in portal hepatic blood flow [19,22,23]. In cats [24] and in baboons [22] fed alcohol chronically, defective oxygen use rather than lack of blood oxygen supply characterized liver injury produced by high concentrations of ethanol. The low oxygen tension normally prevailing in perivenular zones exaggerates the redox shift produced by ethanol [19]. Hypoxia, by increasing NADH, may in turn inhibit the activity of NAD^+-dependent xanthine dehydrogenase, thereby favoring that of oxygen-dependent xanthine oxidase (XO) [25] (Fig. 3). Purine metabolism via XO may lead to the production of oxygen radicals, which can mediate toxic effects toward liver cells, including peroxidation. Physiologic substrates for XO, hypoxanthine, and xanthine, as well as adenosine 5′-monophosphate (adenylic acid, AMP), significantly increased in the liver after ethanol, together with an enhanced urinary output of allantoin (a final product of xanthine metabolism). Allopurinol pretreatment resulted in 90% inhibition of XO activity, and also significantly decreased ethanol-induced lipid peroxidation [25]. Zonal distribution of some enzymes can influence the selective perivenular toxicity. As discussed subsequently, proliferation of the smooth endoplasmic reticulum (SER) after chronic ethanol consumption is maximal in the perivenular zone, with associated enzyme induction and related effects. Furthermore, human ADH predominates in the hepatocytes around the terminal hepatic venule. Thus, a presumably higher level of ethanol metabolism in the perivenular zone could contribute to the increased hepatotoxicity of ethanol, for instance by providing (together with the "induced" microsomal pathway: vide infra) an increased amount of the toxic metabolite acetaldehyde [26]. One must, however, also take into account that after chronic ethanol consumption, ADH may not change or even decreases in activity [27–30], unlike a microsomal ethanol oxidizing system (MEOS), which is induced. Alcoholics may display decreased hepatic ADH activity even in the absence of liver damage [31].

The bulk of hepatic ADH is present in the hepatocytes, but traces are also found in stellate cells [32]. Their role was questioned until Flisiak et al [33] showed that acetaldehyde derived from ADH-mediated ethanol metabolism significantly increases prostanoid production in these rat stellate cells; the presence of ADH has been confirmed in human stellate cells [34].

Pathogenic role of alcohol dehydrogenase polymorphism

Individual differences in the rate of ethanol metabolism may be genetically controlled. Furthermore, genetic factors influence the severity of alcohol-induced liver disease. Indeed, the frequency of an ADH 3 allele has been found to differ in patients with alcohol-related end-organ damage (including cirrhosis) and matched controls, suggesting that genetically determined differences in alcohol metabolism may explain differences in the susceptibility to alcohol-related disease (possibly through the enhanced generation of toxic metabolites) [35], but this hypothesis has been questioned [36].

Microsomal ethanol oxidizing system

Characterization of the microsomal ethanol oxidizing system and its role in ethanol metabolism

   Although recognized only 36 years ago, this new pathway has been the subject of extensive research, reviewed in detail elsewhere [37]. The first indication of an interaction of ethanol with the microsomal fraction of the hepatocyte was provided by the morphologic observation that alcohol feeding results in a proliferation of the SER both in rats [38,39] and in humans [14]. This increase in SER resembles that seen after the administration of a wide variety of hepatotoxins [40], therapeutic agents [41], and some food additives [42]. Because most of the substances that induce a proliferation of the SER are metabolized, at least in part, by the cytochrome P-450 enzyme system that is located on the SER, the possibility that alcohol may also be metabolized by similar enzymes was raised. Such a system was indeed demonstrated in liver microsomes in vitro and found to be inducible by chronic alcohol feeding in vivo [43], and was named the MEOS [29,43]. Its distinct nature was shown by [44] isolation of a P-450-containing fraction from liver microsomes which, although devoid of any ADH or cata-lase activity, could still oxidize ethanol as well as higher aliphatic alcohols (eg, butanol, which is not a substrate for catalase) [45,46] and [47] reconstitution of ethanol-oxidizing activity using NADPH-cytochrome P-450 reductase, phospholipid, and either partially purified or highly purified microsomal P-450 from untreated [48] or phenobarbital-treated [49] rats. That chronic ethanol consumption results in the induction of a unique P-450 was shown by Ohnishi and Lieber [48] using a liver microsomal P-450 fraction isolated from ethanol-treated rats. An ethanol-inducible form of P-450, purified from rabbit liver microsomes [50], catalyzed ethanol oxidation at rates much higher than other P-450 isozymes, and also had an enhanced capacity to oxidize 1-butanol, 1-pen-tanol, and aniline [51], acetaminophen [52], CCl_4 [51], acetone [53], and N-nitrosodimethylamine (NDMA) [54]. The purified protein (now called CYP2E1) was obtained in a catalytically active form, with a high turnover rate for ethanol and other specific substrates [55]. MEOS has a relatively high K_m for ethanol (8–10 mM, compared with 0.2–2 mM for hepatic ADH) but, contrasting with hepatic ADH, which is not inducible in primates as well as most other animal species, enhanced levels of both hepatic 2E1 protein and mRNA were found in actively-drinking patients [56].

   The presence of CYP2E1 was also shown in extrahepatic tissues [57] and in nonparenchymal cells of the liver, including Kupffer [58] but not stellate [34] cells.

Polymorphism of CYP2E1

   Several polymorphic sites in the 5′-flanking region of the human cytochrome *2E1* gene have been reported. Indeed, it contains several restriction fragment-length polymorphisms that may affect transcriptional regulation or the functional activity of the expressed protein [59–63]. Two nucleotide exchanges are within restriction sites (*Pst*I and *Rsa*I) and were found to be in complete linkage disequilibrium. The *Rsa*I sites in the regulatory 5′-flanking region described in Japanese subjects were found to affect the rate of transcription when coupled to a reporter gene in an in vitro expression system [59,63]. Hayashi et al [59] classified the genotypes as type A (homozygous "normal" alleles; *c1,c1*), type C (homozygous alleles with the nucleotide exchanges; *c2,c2*) and type B (hetero-zygous, having a normal and an altered allele; *c1,c2*). The rare mutant allele (termed the *c2* allele) that lacks the *Rsa*I restriction site is associated with higher transcriptional activity, protein levels, and enzyme activity than the more com-mon wild-type allele (*c1* allele) [59,63,64].

The frequency of the *Rsa*I-lacking *c2* allele varies in different populations [65]. The highest frequency has been observed in the Taiwanese (0.28) and Japanese (0.19–0.27), while in African Americans, European Americans, and Scandinavians, the frequency is much lower, ranging between 0.01 and 0.05 [65]. The *Rsa*I polymorphism has been investigated in the Japanese population by two groups: one study showed a positive association of the *c2* allele with alcoholic liver disease [66], while the other study showed an association between the *c1* (wild-type) allele and alcoholic liver disease [67]. A smaller study has also been performed in North American Caucasian men [68]; it did not show an association between alcoholic liver disease and the *Rsa*I polymorphism, whereas Pirmohamed et al [69] found that the *c2* allele frequency in patients with alcoholic liver disease was significantly higher than in control subjects. The discrepancies between the different studies may be related to clinical dissimi-larities of the patients investigated as well as to differences in the gene frequencies of the populations studied. Polymorphism of *CYP2E1* may also play an important role in cigarette smoking-related hepatocarcinogenesis. In a recent, as yet unconfirmed, study a much greater risk was observed for those smokers who were also habitual alcohol drinkers and carried the *c1/c1* genotype [70]. However, *Rsa*I polymorphism did not affect lung cancer risk [71].

*Dra*I polymorphism of *2E1* has been reported to be associated with lung cancer risk in Japanese [62]. However, observations in the United States [72], Finland [60], and Brazil [73] have not supported these findings. There was also no significant difference in *c2* gene frequency between alcoholic and non-alcoholic controls [74]. Similarly, Maezawa et al [75] found no significant difference in the frequency of the *CYP2E1* genotype between alcoholics and healthy subjects, concluding that polymorphisms of the gene does not influence the risk of developing alcoholism in Japanese.

Role of cytochromes P-450 other than CYP2E1

Despite the discovery of CYP2E1 and its prevailing role in microsomal ethanol oxidation, the term MEOS was maintained because cytochromes P-450 other than CYP2E1, as well as hydroxy radicals, can contribute to ethanol metabolism in the microsomes. Indeed, in rat liver microsomes, ethanol is oxidized not only by CYP2E1 but also by CYP1A2 [76]. In humans also, there were some indications of the involvement of P-450s other than CYP2E1 [55].

Specifically, it was demonstrated that human CYP2E1 and CYP1A2 (expressed in β-lymphoblastoid cells) can oxidize ethanol [77]. Furthermore, human CYP2E1, CYP1A2, and CYP3A4 were heterologously expressed in HepG2 cells, and their ethanol oxidation was assessed using corresponding selective inhibitors [78]. All three P-450 isoenzymes metabolized ethanol. Selective inhibitors also decreased microsomal ethanol oxidation in the livers of 18 organ donors. The P-450-dependent ethanol oxidizing activities correlated significantly with those of the specific monooxygenases and the immunochemically determined microsomal content of the respective P-450. The mean CYP2E1-dependent ethanol oxidation was twice that of CYP1A2 or CYP3A4. Thus, CYP2E1 plays the major role in the ethanol oxidation by human liver microsomes, but because the combined activity of CYP1A2 and CYP3A4 is comparable to that of CYP2E1, these P-450s can significantly contribute to microsomal ethanol oxidation and may, therefore, also be involved in related pathophysiology.

Nutritional role of CYP2E1

CYP2E1 is inducible by fasting in the rat [79]. The increase may be due, at least in part, to ketones. Indeed, in rats [80], rabbits [81], and humans [82], acetone appears to be actively used, being metabolized by a microsomal acetone monooxygenase identified as CYP2E1 [83,84]. Acetone is both an inducer and a substrate of CYP2E1 [85,86]. The existence of a gluconeogenic pathway for acetone was shown by the incorporation of [^{14}C] acetone into glucose and amino acids during fasting and diabetic ketoacidosis [82,87,88] accounting for 10% of the gluconeogenic demands. The conversion of acetone to acetol and then to methylglyoxal, both intermediates in the gluconeogenic pathway, was demonstrated in vitro [80,81]. The contribution of CYP2E1 to the biotransformation of acetone was also shown in vivo by the increase in blood acetone after the CYP2E1 inhibitors diallyl sulfide, diallyl sulfoxide, and diallyl sulfone [89].

The activity of CYP2E1 in fatty acid metabolism also illustrates the nutritional role for CYP2E1. Indeed, CYP2E1, in addition to its ethanol oxidizing activity, catalyzes fatty acid ω-1 and ω-2 hydroxylations [90–92]. As mentioned, ethanol feeding also results in an increased activity of CYP4A1 [93], and this CYP4A subfamily catalyzes ω-hydroxylation at the terminal carbon of fatty acids.

Role of microsomal ethanol oxidizing system and associated cytochromes P-450 in hepatic and extra hepatic pathology

The mechanisms whereby alcohol causes liver injury are still not fully elucidated. However, in a recent study on CYP2E1 induction among alcoholics it was reported that the oxidation of chlorzoxazone, a CYP2E1 substrate, was significantly higher in patients with liver injury than in alcoholics without clinical and biochemical signs of liver disease [94], which suggests a link between the two. Indeed, polyenylphosphatidylcholine (PPC) and its active component dilinoleoylphosphatidylcholine (DLPC) were found to decrease CYP2E1 activity [95,96]. Furthermore, PPC was discovered to oppose oxidative stress [97] and fibrosis [98] in alcohol-fed baboons. Thus, much of the medical significance of MEOS (and its ethanol-inducible CYP2E1) results not only from the oxidation of ethanol but also from the unusual and unique capacity of CYP2E1 to generate reactive oxygen intermediates, such as superoxide radicals (Fig. 3) [99], and to activate many xenobiotic compounds to their toxic metabolites, often free radicals. This pertains, for instance, to carbon tetrachloride and other industrial solvents such as bromobenzene [100], and vinylidene chloride [101], as well as anesthetics such as enflurane [102], and halothane [103]. Ethanol also markedly increased the activity of microsomal low K_m benzene metabolizing enzymes [104] and aggravated the hemopoietic toxicity of benzene. Enhanced metabolism (and toxicity) pertains also to a variety of prescribed drugs, including isoniazid and phenylbutazone [105] and some over-the-counter medications such as acetaminophen (paracetamol, N-acetyl-p-aminophenol), all of which are substrates for, or inducers of, CYP2E1. Therapeutic amounts of acetaminophen (2.5 to 4 g/d) can cause hepatic injury in alcoholics. In animals given ethanol for long periods, hepatotoxic effects peak after withdrawal [106] when ethanol is no longer competing for the microsomal pathway but levels of the toxic metabolites are at their highest. Thus, alcoholics are most vulnerable to the toxic effects of acetaminophen shortly after cessation of chronic drinking. In fact, such patients hospitalized with acetaminophen toxicity related to accidental misuse had higher rates of morbidity and mortality than those who attempted suicide, even though the latter had taken more acetaminophen [107].

There is an association between alcohol misuse and an increased incidence of upper alimentary and respiratory tract cancers [108]. Many factors have been incriminated; one of which is the effect of ethanol on enzyme systems involved CYP-dependent activation of carcinogens. This effect has been demonstrated with the use of microsomes derived from a variety of tissues, including the liver (the principal site of xenobiotic metabolism) [109,110], the lungs [109,110], and intestines [57,111] (the chief portals of entry for tobacco smoke and dietary carcinogens, respectively), as well as esophagus [112] (where ethanol consumption is a major risk factor in the development of cancer). Alcoholics are commonly heavy smokers, and a synergistic effect of alcohol consumption and smoking on cancer development has been described, as reviewed elsewhere [108]. Indeed, long-term ethanol consumption was found to enhance the mutagenicity of tobacco-derived products [108]. Alcohol may also influence carcinogenesis in many other ways [113], one of which involves vitamin A depletion (vide infra).

There is increased evidence that ethanol toxicity may be associated with an increased production of reactive oxygen intermediates. Numerous experimental data indicate that free radical mechanisms contribute to ethanol-induced liver injury. Increased generation of oxygen- and ethanol-derived free radicals occur at the microsomal level, especially through the intervention of the ethanol-inducible CYP2E1 (Fig. 3) [114]. This induction is associated with proliferation of the endoplasmic reticulum (vide supra), which is accompanied by increased oxidation of NADPH with resulting H_2O_2 generation [29]. There is also increased superoxide radical production. In addition, the CYP2E1 induction contributes to the well-known lipid peroxidation associated with alcoholic liver injury. DiLuzio [115,116] was one of the first to report that ethanol produces increased lipid peroxidation in the liver, and that the ethanol-induced fatty liver could be prevented by antioxidants. Lipid peroxidation correlated with the amount of CYP2E1 in liver microsomal preparations, and it could be inhibited by antibodies against CYP2E1 in control and ethanol-fed rats [117,118]. Indeed, CYP2E1 is rather "leaky," and its operation results in a significant release of free radicals, including l-hydroxyethyl free radical intermediates [119,120], confirmed by detecting the hydroxyethyl radicals in vivo [121].

Ethanol can also be reduced by liver microsomes to acetaldehyde through a nonenzymatic pathway involving the presence of hydroxyl radicals originating from iron-catalyzed degradation of H_2O_2 [122]. The production of ethanol-free radicals may be due to an oxidizing species bound to cytochrome P-450 and abstracting a proton from the alcohol α-carbon [123] in catalyzing the free radical activation of aliphatic alcohols. Biochem Pharmacol, 411:1895, 1991.]. It is not known, however, whether hydroxyethyl free radicals contribute to the damaging effects of ethanol. Hydroxyethyl radicals appear to be involved in the alkylation of hepatic proteins. In vitro produced hydroxyethyl radical forms stable adducts with albumin or fibrinogen [124] and patients with alcoholic cirrhosis have increased serum levels of both IgG and IgA reacting with proteins of liver microsomes incubated with ethanol and NADPH [124], which do not crossreact with the epitopes derived from acetaldehyde-modified proteins.

Most importantly, induction of the MEOS results in enhanced acetaldehyde production which, in turn, aggravates the oxidative stress directly and as well as indirectly, by impairing defense systems against it (vide infra).

Toxic interactions of ethanol with retinol and β-carotene

Already at early stages of alcoholic liver disease, there is severe associated hepatic vitamin A depletion [125]. Experimentally, depressed hepatic levels of vitamin A were observed even when alcohol was given with diets containing large amounts of vitamin A [126]. Hepatic vitamin A depletion is associated with lysosomal lesions [127] and decreased detoxification of NDMA [128]. New hepatic pathways of retinol metabolism have been discovered [129,130] and, because these enzymes are inducible by either ethanol or drug administration, they contribute to the depletion.

Not only does vitamin A deficiency adversely affect the liver [127], but an excess of vitamin A is also known to be hepatotoxic [131]. Long-term ethanol consumption enhances this effect, resulting in striking morphologic and functional alterations of the mitochondria [132], along with hepatic necrosis and fibrosis [133]. Hypervitaminosis A itself can induce fibrosis and even cirrhosis, as reviewed elsewhere [132]. Thus, alcohol abuse narrows the therapeutic window for vitamin A, thereby hindering its therapeutic use.

In contrast to retinoids, carotenoids (even when ingested chronically in large amounts) were not known to produce toxic manifestations [134,135]. Therefore, it made sense to assess whether carotenoids may serve as effective (but less toxic) substitutes for retinol, especially in alcoholic liver injury that has been attributed, in part, to oxidative stress and because β-carotene is an antioxidant. Indeed, studies by Mobarhan et al [136] showed that replenishing young men with β-carotene can decrease the level of circulating lipid peroxides, but it was not reported whether this can be achieved in individuals who continue to drink and at a dose of β-carotene that has no toxicity in the presence of alcohol. Indeed, in the studies of Mobarhan et al [136], the subjects had stopped taking alcohol at the time they received the β-carotene. The question therefore remained as to whether the combination of alcohol and β-carotene, at the dose used for replenishment, may be useful in terms of preventing lipid peroxidation, without producing some signs of toxicity.

Studies in humans revealed that for a given β-carotene intake, there is a correlation between alcohol consumption and plasma β-carotene concentration [47]. Thus, whereas in general, alcoholics have low plasma β-carotene levels [47,137], presumably reflecting low intake, alcohol per se might, in fact, increase blood levels in humans [37]. There was also an increase in women (with a dose as low as two drinks a day [138], and also in nonhuman primates [139]. Indeed, in baboons fed ethanol chronically, liver β-carotene was increased, in contrast with vitamin A, which was depleted. Similarly, plasma β-carotene levels were elevated in ethanol-fed baboons, with a striking delay in the clearance from the blood after a β-carotene load. Furthermore, whereas β-carotene administration increased hepatic vitamin A in control baboons, this effect was much less evident in alcohol-fed animals. The combination of an increase in β-carotene and a relative lack of a corresponding rise in vitamin A suggests a blockage in the conversion of β-carotene to vitamin A by ethanol.

The relationship between liver disease and hepatic carotenoids is complex. In most patients with liver disease, absolute levels of hepatic α- and β-carotene and retinoids were found to be severely depressed, even in the presence of normal serum levels of lycopene α and-or β-carotene; in patients with cirrhosis, hepatic levels were particularly low [140]. However, even in these patients with very low liver α- and β-carotene concentrations, more than half had blood levels in the normal range, suggesting that liver disease interferes with the uptake, excretion, or perhaps metabolism of α- and β-carotene. In only one third of the subjects were α- and β-carotene serum levels low, probably reflecting poor dietary intake.

In the baboon, the administration of ethanol together with β-carotene resulted in a more striking hepatic injury than with either compound alone [139]. In the rat also, the well-known hepatotoxicity of ethanol was potentiated by large amounts of β-carotene, and the concomitant administration of both resulted in striking liver lesions [141]. These were characterized at the biochemical level by increased activity of liver enzymes in the plasma, at the light microscopic level by an inflammatory response and, at the ultrastructural level, by striking autophagic vacuoles and alterations of the endoplasmic reticulum and the mitochondria [141]. In the latter study, β-carotene was administered in beadlets, which enhanced its bioavailability. Moreover, beadlets resulted in proliferation of the

SER and in leakage of the mitochondrial glutamate dehydrogenase into the plasma, reflecting mitochondrial injury (both documented by electron microscopy) [141].

In addition, some extrahepatic side effects were observed. It was noted that in smokers, β-carotene supplementation increased death from coronary heart disease (ATBC Study [44] and CARET Trial [142]).

The toxic effects of β-carotene and their interaction with ethanol also involve an increased incidence of pulmonary cancer. Both the ATBC [44] and the CARET [142] studies, revealed that β-carotene supplementation increases the incidence of pulmonary cancer in smokers. Because heavy smokers are commonly heavy drinkers, we raised the possibility that alcohol abuse was contributory [143]. Indeed, it was subsequently shown that the increased incidence of pulmonary cancer was related to the alcohol consumed [144,145].

The catalase pathway

Catalase is capable of oxidizing alcohol in vitro in the presence of an H_2O_2-generating system [146] (Fig. 3) and its interaction with H_2O_2 in the intact liver was demonstrated [147]. However, its role is limited by the small amount of H_2O_2 generated [48] and, under physiologic conditions, catalase thus appears to play no major role in ethanol oxidation.

The catalase contribution might be enhanced if significant amounts of H_2O_2 become available through β-oxidation of fatty acids in peroxisomes [148]. However, the peroxisomal enzymes do not oxidize short-chain fatty acids such as octanoate, and peroxisomal β-oxidation was observed only in the absence of ADH activity. In its presence, the rate of ethanol metabolism is reduced by adding fatty acids [149]. and, conversely, β-oxidation of fatty acids is inhibited by NADH produced from ethanol metabolism via ADH [149]. Similarly, generation of reducing equivalents from ethanol by ADH in the cytosol inhibits H_2O_2 generation leading to significantly diminished rates of peroxidation of alcohols via catalase [150]. Various other results also indicated that peroxisomal fatty acid oxidation does not play a major role in alcohol metabolism [151]. Furthermore, when fatty acids were used by Handler and Thurman [148] to stimulate ethanol oxidation, this effect was very sensitive to inhibition by aminotriazole, a catalase inhibitor. Therefore, if this mechanism were to play an important role in vivo, one would expect a significant inhibition of ethanol metabolism after aminothiazole administration in vivo, when physiologic amounts of fatty acids and other substrates for H_2O_2 generation are present. A number of studies, however, have shown that aminotriazole treatment has a little, if any, effect on alcohol oxidation in vivo [103,152,153] Despite the considerable controversy that originally surrounded this issue, it is now agreed by the principal contenders involved that catalase cannot account for microsomal ethanol oxidation [46,154]. However, catalase could contribute to fatty acid oxidation. Indeed, long-term ethanol consumption is associated with increases in the content of a specific cytochrome (CYP4A1) that promotes microsomal ω-hydroxylation of fatty acids that may compensate, at least in part, for the deficit in fatty acid oxidation due to the

ethanol induced injury of the mitochondria [155] (Abstract)]. Products of
ω-oxidation also increase liver cytosolic fatty acid-binding protein content and
peroxisomal β-oxidation [156], an alternate but modest pathway for fatty acid
disposition (vide supra).

*Acetaldehyde metabolism and toxicity, including glutathione depletion and
lipid peroxidation*

Acetaldehyde, the product of ethanol oxidation, is highly toxic and rapidly
metabolized to acetate, mainly by a mitochondrial low K_m aldehyde dehydrogenase (ALDH2), the activity of which is lacking in about 25% to 50% of Orientals.
In these individuals, even small amounts of alcohol that have almost no effect
on Caucasians can produce a rapid facial flush, frequently associated with
tachycardia, headache, and nausea [157]. This propensity for flushing is genetically determined and caused by decreased disposition secondary to the lack of
ALDH2 activity [158–161]. In fact, the flushing reaction seen in susceptible
Orientals mimics to a lesser degree the disulfiram reaction caused by the
elevation of acetaldehyde following aldehyde dehydrogenase inhibition. This
reaction has gained widespread therapeutic use as a reinforcement for abstinence
in alcoholism rehabilitation programs. Actually, the aversive cardiovascular
effects of acetaldehyde may contribute to the relatively lower incidence of
cirrhosis in "flushers" [162]. The flushing phenotype may also confer some
resistance to the development of alcoholism [163]. Conversely, however,
Japanese alcoholics with an ALDH2 deficiency and, presumably, higher hepatic
acetaldehyde levels during drinking, developed alcoholic liver disease at a lower
cumulative intake of ethanol than a control group [164].

The ALDH activity is also significantly reduced by chronic ethanol
consumption [165]. The decreased capacity of mitochondria of alcohol-fed
subjects to oxidize acetaldehyde, associated with unaltered or even enhanced
rates of ethanol oxidation (and therefore acetaldehyde generation because of
MEOS induction: vide supra) results in an imbalance between production and
disposition of acetaldehyde. The latter causes the elevated acetaldehyde levels
observed after chronic ethanol consumption in humans [166] and in baboons,
which revealed a tremendous increase of acetaldehyde in hepatic venous blood
[22], reflecting high tissue levels.

Acetaldehyde's toxicity is due, in part, to its capacity to form protein adducts,
resulting in antibody production, enzyme inactivation, and decreased DNA repair
[22,167]. It is also associated with a striking impairment of the capacity of
the liver to use oxygen. Moreover, acetaldehyde promotes glutathione (GSH)
depletion, free radical-mediated toxicity, and lipid peroxidation. Indeed,
acetaldehyde was shown to be capable of causing lipid peroxidation in isolated
perfused livers [168,169]. In vitro, metabolism of acetaldehyde via XO or
aldehyde oxidase may generate free radicals, but the concentration of acetaldehyde required is much too high for this mechanism to be of significance in
vivo. However, another mechanism to promote lipid peroxidation is via GSH

depletion. One of the three amino acids of this tripeptide is cysteine. Binding of acetaldehyde with cysteine or GSH may contribute to a depression of liver GSH [170]. Rats fed ethanol chronically have significantly increased rates of GSH turnover [171]. Acute ethanol administration inhibits GSH synthesis and produces an increased loss from the liver [172]. GSH is selectively depleted in the mitochondria [173], and may contribute to the striking alcohol-induced alterations of that organelle. GSH offers one of the mechanisms for the scavenging of toxic free radicals, as shown in Fig. 4, which also illustrates how the ensuing enhanced GSH use (and thus turnover) results in a significant increase in α-amino-*n*-butyric acid [21]. Although GSH depletion per se may not be sufficient to cause lipid peroxidation, it is generally agreed upon that it may favor the peroxidation produced by other factors. GSH has been shown to spare and potentiate vitamin E [174]; it is important in the protection of cells against electrophilic drug injury in general, and against reactive oxygen species in particular, especially in primates, which are more vulnerable to GSH depletion than rodents [175]. Iron overload may play a contributory role, because chronic alcohol consumption results in increased iron uptake by hepatocytes [176], and because iron exposure accentuates the changes of lipid peroxidation and in the GSH status of the liver cell induced by acute ethanol intoxication [177]. It is also of interest that genetic factors may play a role. There is an apparent association between the occurrence of GSH-S-transferase M1 "null" genotype and alcoholic liver disease, the "null" genotype indicating absent activity of class μ GSH transferase [178]. Other genetic factors have also been implicated: in addition to the ALDH2 deficiency and the CYP2E polymorphism (vide supra), a significant

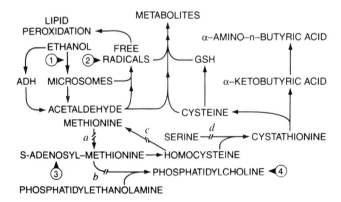

Fig. 4. Lipid peroxidation and other consequences of alcoholic liver disease or increased free radical generation and acetaldehyde production by ethanol-induced microsomes, with sites of new therapeutic interventions. Metabolic blocks caused by liver disease (*a,b*), folate (*c*), B12 (*c*) or B6 (*d*) deficiencies are illustrated, with corresponding depletions in SAMe, phosphatidylcholine, and GSH. New therapeutic approaches include (1) downregulation of microsomal enzyme induction especially of CYP2E1, (2) decrease of free radicals, with antioxidants (3) replenishment of SAMe and of (4) phosphatidylcholine (*From* Lieber CS. Alcoholic liver disease: new insights in pathogenesis lead to new treatments. J Hepatol 2000;32:113–28; with permission.)

association, with alcoholic cirrhosis, of a particular restriction fragment length polymorphism haplotype of the COL1A2 locus of the collagen type I gene has been reported by Weiner et al [179] but questioned by others [180].

Correction of the alcohol-induced oxidative stress in the liver

All the pathways of ethanol oxidation result in oxidative stress and associated lipid peroxidation, either directly or through the product acetaldehyde. However, lipid peroxidation is not only a reflection of tissue damage, but it may also play a pathogenic role by promoting collagen production [181,182]. The ADH-mediated redox damage also stimulates expression of collagen [34]. Thus, correction of oxidative stress is becoming central to efforts at prevention.

Methionine and S-adenosyl methionine

As already mentioned, one major antioxidant agent depleted by ethanol and acetaldehyde is the reduced form of GSH. However, therapeutic use of GSH itself is complicated by the fact that its replenishment through supplementation is hampered by its poor penetration into the hepatocytes, except for the ethyl derivative, which of course is not very suitable for the treatment of alcoholic liver injury. Cysteine is one of the three amino acids of GSH, and the ultimate precursor of cysteine is methionine (Fig. 4); its deficiency in alcoholics has been incriminated, and its supplementation has been considered for the treatment of alcoholic liver injury, but some difficulties have been encountered. Indeed, excess methionine was shown to have some adverse effects [183], including a decrease in hepatic ATP. Horowitz et al [184], reported that the blood clearance of methionine after an oral load of this amino acid was slowed in patients with cirrhosis. Because about half the methionine is metabolized by the liver, the above observations suggest impaired hepatic metabolism of this amino acid in patients with alcoholic liver disease. Indeed, to be used, methionine has to be activated to S-adenosylmethionine (SAMe) (Fig. 4), but Duce et al [185] found a decrease in SAMe synthetase activity in cirrhotic livers, now linked to the regulation of methionine adenosyltransferase activity and gene expression by hypoxia. Nitric oxide-mediated inactivation and transcriptional arrest seem to be the two major pathways by which oxygen levels control hepatic SAMe syn-thetase activity [186]. As a consequence, SAMe depletion ensues after chronic ethanol consumption [187]. Potentially, such SAMe depletion, may have a number of adverse effects. In addition to trapping free radicals via GSH (Fig. 4), SAMe is the principal methylating agent in various transmethylation reactions important for nucleic acid and protein synthesis, as well as membrane fluidity and functions, including the transport of metabolites and transmission of signals across membranes and maintenance of membranes. In addition, SAMe plays a key role in the synthesis of polyamines. Thus, depletion of SAMe may promote the membrane injury documented in alcohol-induced liver damage [188].

Compared with methionine, administration of SAMe has the advantage of bypassing the deficit in SAMe synthesis (from methionine) referred to above

(Fig. 4). The usefulness of SAMe administration has been shown in the baboon [187] and in various clinical studies [189,190], including the demonstration that it significantly decreases the mortality in patients with alcoholic cirrhosis [191].

Polyenyl- and dilinoleoyl-phosphatidylcholine

It is generally believed that polyunsaturated lipids favor peroxidation because of their multiple double-bond configuration, which renders them more susceptible than saturated or monounsaturated ones to free radical peroxidation [192]. Surprisingly, however, evidence gathered in rodents and in nonhuman primates revealed striking antioxidant effects of a soybean extract rich in polyunsaturated lecithin, namely PPC, about half of which consists of DLPC [98]. It was found that PPC prevents hepatic lipid peroxidation and attenuates associated injury induced by CCl_4 in rats [193]. Furthermore, PPC also decreased oxidant stress in the baboon [97,155], a species in which protection by PPC against alcohol-induced liver injury (including fibrosis and cirrhosis) was also previously mentioned [98].

Using gas chromatography/mass spectroscopy (GC/MS), hepatic OH-nonenal, and F_2-isoprostanes, parameters of lipid peroxidation, were determined in liver needle biopsies. Whereas alcohol increased both, PPC administration resulted in their significant reduction, and it also attenuated the alcohol-induced decrease in GSH [97].

As the phospholipid species of PPC are highly bioavailable (vide infra) and readily integrated in the liver membranes, they could scavenge the excess O_2 free radicals and thereby prevent their toxic interaction with critical membrane polyunsaturated fatty acids. In a sense, they could act as some kind of radical "trap" or "sink" [194].

Furthermore, because peroxidation products are fibrogenic [181,182], their decrease after PPC could also explain, at least in part, the antifibrogenic property of the phospholipids.

PPC may also restore key enzyme activity. Indeed, the impairment of the mitochondria after chronic ethanol consumption includes a significant decrease in cytochrome oxidase activity, associated with a depletion in mitochondrial phosphatidylcholine; replenishment of the latter restored the cytochrome oxidase activity in vitro [195]. One of the key functions of phosphatidylethanol-amine methyltransferase (PEMT) is to use SAMe as a methyl donor in the methylation of phosphatidylethylanolamine to phosphatidylcholine (Fig. 4). However, chronic ethanol consumption is associated with a decrease of this enzyme activity, both in baboons [196] and in humans [185]. The decrease in PEMT activity after alcohol may have some secondary effects on liver phospholipids. Indeed, it may be responsible, at least in part, for the associated decrease in phospholipids [98,196]. Supplementation with PPC was shown to restore the PEMT activity [196]. Thus, on the one hand, PEMT depletion after alcohol may exacerbate the hepatic phospholipid depletion and the associated membrane abnormalities, thereby promoting hepatic injury and triggering fibrosis, whereas PPC, by repleting hepatic phospholipids and normalizing PEMT activity, may contribute to the protection against alcoholic cirrhosis provided by PPC supplementation [98,196,197].

PPC is especially suited to correct hepatic phospholipid depletion because it has a high bioavailability. More than 50% of orally administered PPC is made biologically available for the organism either by intact absorption (lesser extent) or by reacylation of absorbed lysophosphatidyl-choline (greater extent) [198]. Supplementation with PPC, which is rich in DLPC, results in an increase, in the liver, of DLPC, which may be the active compound. Indeed, in cultured stellate cells, PPC prevented the acetaldehyde-mediated collagen accumulation [199], at least in part, by stimulating collagenase activity, the latter effect was fully duplicated by DLPC [98].

The hepatoprotective effect of PPC was manifest not only for the prevention, but also for the attenuation of preexisting liver fibrosis and cirrhosis [200]. Furthermore, PPC acts at prefibrotic steps: it attenuated hepatomegaly, fatty liver, and hyperlipemia in alcohol-fed rats [201].

Vitamin E and other antioxidants

Bjørneboe et al [202] reported a reduced hepatic α-tocopherol content after chronic ethanol feeding in rats receiving adequate amounts of vitamin E, as well as in the blood of alcoholics. Hepatic lipid peroxidation was also significantly increased after chronic ethanol feeding in rats receiving a low vitamin E diet [203], indicating that dietary vitamin E is an important determinant of hepatic lipid peroxidation induced by chronic ethanol feeding. The lowest hepatic α-tocopherol was found in rats receiving a combination of low vitamin E and ethanol: both low dietary vitamin E and ethanol feeding significantly decreased hepatic α-tocopherol content, the latter, in part, because of increased conversion of α-tocopherol to α-tocopherylquinone [203]. In patients with cirrhosis, diminished hepatic vitamin E levels have been observed [204,205]. Effectiveness of vitamin E supplementation in the prevention of alcoholic liver injury is presently being evaluated.

Other antioxidant medications that have been proposed include (+)-cyanidanol-3, silymarin, selenium, and thioctic acid, but their beneficial effects still need confirmation [206].

Extrahepatic ethanol metabolism

Oxidation of ethanol in the stomach; gender and ethnic differences

Extrahepatic metabolism of ethanol is low, except for the stomach, which is exposed to high ethanol concentrations that can support the activities of enzymes requiring such levels (such as ADH class IV and V). Alcohol was known to disappear from the stomach, and this was considered to be part of its "absorption" from the gastrointestinal tract. It was quantitated postprandially by Cortot et al [207] in seven healthy subjects. They found that of the ingested alcohol, $39.4 \pm 4.1\%$ was absorbed through the stomach wall during the first postprandial hour and $73.2 \pm 4.2\%$ during the remaining time. It is now apparent that some of this absorbed ethanol is actually metabolized in the gastric wall.

It was also known that when alcohol is taken orally, blood levels achieved are generally lower than those obtained after administration of the same dose intravenously [208,209], the so-called first-pass metabolism (FPM). Many drugs undergo FPM, which usually reflects metabolism in the liver. However, several observations had shown that the gastric mucosa also contains enzymes with ADH activity. The histochemical observations of Pestallozi et al [210] showed that the majority of superficial mucosa cells in the stomach had significant amounts of such activity. In fact, the human gastric mucosa possesses several ADH isoenzymes [211], one of which is a class IV ADH (now called sigma-ADH) and is not present in the liver (Fig. 2). This enzyme has now been purified [212], its full-length cDNA obtained, and the complete amino acid sequence deduced [213,214]. Furthermore, a nearly full-length gene (*ADH7*) was cloned by Satre et al [215]; the full-length gene was obtained by Yokoyama et al [216] and localized to chromosome 4. The upstream structure of human *ADH7* gene and the organ distribution of its expression was also defined [217]. Sigma-ADH was found to have a high capacity for ethanol oxidation, greater than that of the other isozymes. Its affinity for ethanol is relatively low, with a K_m of about 30 mM [212], but this is not a draw back in the stomach where ethanol is commonly present at much higher concentrations.

In vitro, gastric ADH was found to be responsible for a large part of ethanol metabolism found in cultured rat [218] and human [219] gastric cells. However, the in vivo relative contribution of gastric and hepatic ADH to ethanol metabolism has been the subject of debate [220–223], but studies of Lim et al [224] showed true gastric FPM in experiments using the same dose of alcohol given by either intragastric intubation or by intravenous, intraportal, and intraduodenal infusions at a rate that mimicked the loss of alcohol from the stomach. Furthermore, rats that had developed portosystemic shunts after ligation of the portal vein exhibited blood alcohol curves and FPM equivalent to those of sham-operated controls, indicating again that FPM is not dependent on first-pass flow through the liver, but reflects, at least in part, gastric metabolism [224].

The concept of ethanol metabolism in the stomach was also supported indirectly by the observation that commonly used drugs, such as aspirin [225], and some H_2-blockers [211,226], which decrease the activity of gastric ADH [211,218,219,226,227] or accelerate gastric emptying [228], also increased blood alcohol levels in vivo. This was particularly apparent after repeated intake of low alcohol doses, mimicking social drinking (Fig. 5). Although questioned at first, such increases in blood levels have now been confirmed [229,230] for low ethanol doses. The blood level achieved by each single administration of such low doses is small, but social drinking is usually characterized by repetitive consumption of such small doses. Under those conditions, the effect of the drug is cumulative [231] (Fig. 5), and the increase in blood alcohol becomes sufficient to reach levels known to impair cognitive and fine motor functions [232–234].

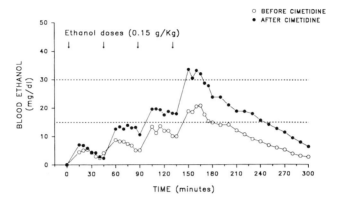

Fig. 5. Effects of cimetidine (400 mg twice a day for 7 days) on average blood alcohol levels after oral consumption of ethanol in nine subjects. Four small doses of ethanol (150 mg/k) were imbibed at 45-minute intervals, before and after administration of cimetidine. The effect of cimetidine on repeated drinking was significant ($P<0.01$ by two-way analysis of variance for repeated measures) (*From* Gupta AM, Baraona E, Lieber CS. Significant increase of blood alcohol by cimetidine after repetitive drinking of small alcohol doses. Alcohol Clin Exp Res 1995;19:1083–7.)

Some ethnic differences also support the concept of the role of gastric ADH in FPM of ethanol. Indeed, sigma-ADH is absent or markedly decreased in activity in a large percentage of Japanese subjects [235]. Their FPM is reduced correspondingly [236], in keeping with a predominant role for sigma-ADH in human FPM. Thus, the FPM represents some kind of "protective barrier" against the systemic effects of ethanol, and its stimulation was invoked to explain some associated attenuation of liver damage [237,238].

Gender differences have also been described: women have a greater vulnerability than men to the development of organ damage after chronic alcoholic abuse, both in terms of liver disease [239–242] and brain damage [243]. It is noteworthy that in Caucasians, gastric ADH activity is lower in women than in men [244], at least below the age of 50 years [245]. There was associated higher blood alcohol levels, an effect more striking in alcoholic than in nonalcoholic women [244] because FPM is partly lost in the alcoholic [166], together with decreased gastric ADH activity. Furthermore, in women, the alcohol consumed is distributed in a 12% smaller water space [244] because of a difference in body composition (more fat and less water).

The magnitude of FPM also depends on the concentration of the alcoholic beverages used. Indeed, gastric ADH isozymes require a relatively high ethanol concentration for optimal activity (vide supra). Therefore, the concentration of alcoholic beverages affects the amount metabolized [246], with lesser FPM and higher blood levels after beer than whiskey [247] for equivalent amounts of ethanol. Fasting also strikingly decreases FPM [166], most likely because of accelerated gastric emptying, resulting in shortened exposure of ethanol to gastric ADH, and its more rapid intestinal absorption. When alcohol is being metabolized in the stomach, it is converted to acetaldehyde, a toxic metabolite, and some resulting gastric injury can be expected. It is possible, of course, that alternatively, or in addition, alcohol may favor gastric injury in some other ways. For instance, the alcohol (or acetaldehyde) induced mucosal injury may, in turn, promote implantation or persistence in the stomach of *Helicobactor pylori* (HP). An increased incidence of HP infection in the alcoholic has been observed [248]. Because both ethanol and the NH_3 generated by HP activate cysteine proteases [249], they also could potentiate each other's gastric toxicity in a similar way and play a role in the pathogenesis of gastritis [250]. Indeed, HP, and hence gastric NH_3, can be eliminated with antibiotics [251,252] and, with the eradication of HP, chronic gastritis usually resolves [253].

Pathologic role of CYP2E1 in Kupffer cells, extrahepatic tissues, and nonalcoholic steatohepatitis

Ethanol affects several Kupffer cell functions that may contribute to the development of alcoholic liver injury, including upregulation of Kuppfer cell CYP2E1 after chronic alcohol consumption [58]. The induction is of the same relative magnitude as in hepatocytes, but in absolute amounts, the CYP2E1 content is 10 times lower than in hepatocytes of the same animals.

The induction of CYP2E1 in Kupffer cells by ethanol has several consequences, including increasing the intracellular levels of acetaldehyde, the toxic metabolite of ethanol. Indeed, Kupffer cells have been shown to metabolize ethanol [254], and the relative contribution of CYP2E1 to overall acetaldehyde production of these cells is probably much higher than in hepatocytes. Indeed, in murine Kupffer cells, cytochrome P-450 inhibitors have been shown to reduce ethanol metabolism by more than 50%, whereas ADH and catalase inhibitors decreased it by less than 10% [254].

Increases of CYP2E1 content of rats fed ethanol with a high-fat diet have been detected in the pancreas by immunohistochemistry [255] and Western blotting [256], but catalytic activity of CYP2E1 in pancreas was not reported initially, probably because of methodologic problems. In a more recent study, improvements in methodology of tissue preparation and enzyme measurements made it possible to detect the CYP2E1 and 1A1 activities in the pancreas and their increase after chronic ethanol treatment [257]. This induction of CYP2E1 and CYP1A1 activities could play a role in the pathogenesis of pancreatitis or pancreatic cancer.

CYP2E1 was also detected on immunoblots of kidney microsomes [258], and it was increased by chronic ethanol treatment [259]. As reviewed before [11], alcohol abuse results in kidney damage, including fat accumulation, which may be linked to the increase of kidney CYP2E1. As reviewed elsewhere [260], CYP2E1 has also been described to a variable extend in a number of other tissues.

As reviewed before, ketones and fatty acids are also substrate and inducer of CYP2E1. Accordingly, in obesity and diabetes, the excess of these substrates commonly results in CYP2E1 upregulation, demonstrated in an experimental model of obesity [261], as well as in patients with nonalcoholic steatohepatitis

(NASH) [262] or in an experimental model of NASH [263]. NASH is increasingly recognized as a precursor to more severe liver disease, leading to "cryptogenic" cirrhosis [264]. In the general population, the prevalence of NAFLD averages 20% and that of NASH 2% to 3% [265]. Thus, these conditions may be the most common liver diseases in the United States. In addition, in view of the pathogenic role that upregulation of CYP2E1 also plays in alcoholic liver disease (vide supra), it is apparent that the major therapeutic challenge is now to find a way to control this toxic process.

Useful physiologic role of CYP2E1

The upregulation of CYP2E1 plays a useful physiologic role when starvation or low-carbohydrate diets prevail because of its contribution to the metabolism of fatty acids and its capacity to convert ketones to glucose [37] (vide supra), and furthermore, although it can activate some xenobiotics to toxic agents as well as carcinogens, it helps detoxify other xenobiotics and it also clears alcohol from the blood when it reaches relatively high levels, particularly when consumed on a chronic basis, which triggers an adaptive CYP2E1 response to the increased substrate concentration, as reviewed elsewhere [260]. However, like many other useful adaptive systems, when the adaptation ceases to be only homeostatic and becomes excessive, adverse consequences prevail. CYP2E1 leaks oxygen radicals as part of its stimulated operation and, when this exceeds the cellular defense systems, it results in oxidative stress, with its various pathologic consequences. This is true not only when excess alcohol has to be metabolized, as is the case in alcoholic steatohepatitis, but also when CYP2E1 is confronted by an excess of ketones and fatty acids associated with diabetes or obesity. These conditions that upregulate CYP2E1 and the resulting oxidative stress generates or aggravates NASH. NASH has been recognized as an important precursor of cryptogenic cirrhosis. The challenge is now to boost the cellular defense systems against oxidative stress as well as to find effective but nontoxic inhibitors of CYP2E1 capable of downregulating its activity.

Nonoxidative metabolism of ethanol

Ethanol can form ethyl esters in vivo, and the corresponding enzyme has been purified [266]. Laposata and Lange [267] have found that, compared with controls, in short-term–intoxicated subjects, concentrations of fatty acid ethyl esters were significantly higher in the pancreas, liver, heart, and adipose tissue. Because in humans this nonoxidative ethanol metabolism occurs in the organs most commonly injured by alcohol abuse, and because some of these organs lack oxidative ethanol metabolism, Laposata and Lange [267] postulated that fatty acid ethyl esters may have a role in the production of alcohol-induced injury. This was corroborated by recent evidence for experimental pancreatic damage [268], but further experiments are needed to verify the possible role of this mechanism in the pathogenesis of alcohol-induced liver injury.

Summary

Alcohol (ethyl alcohol or ethanol) has been associated with mankind since the dawn of civilization, yet its metabolism has only been elucidated in recent years. It had been known since the beginning of the century that catalase, located in the peroxisomes, can break down ethanol, but it is now realized that except for unusual circumstances, this is a minor pathway. The main pathway proceeds via cytosolic ADH, which has multiple isoenzymes, the genetic polymorphism of which is now being unraveled in terms of its possible clinical implications. The latest ADH isozyme to be categorized is sigma-ADH, which is prevalent in the upper gastrointestinal tract and exhibits ethnic variability. Three decades ago, a third and new microsomal pathway of ethanol metabolism was discovered, namely MEOS, which, contrary to the two other pathways, is highly inducible by chronic alcohol consumption. It plays a significant role in alcohol-related pathology through the increased production of the toxic metabolite acetaldehyde, the concomitant generation of free radicals and the cross induction of other microsomal enzymes, especially other cytochromes P-450. These, in turn, activate scores of xenobiotics to highly toxic and carcinogenic metabolites, while contributing to the degradation (hence, the depletion) of vitamin A, and the toxicity of excess retinol and β-carotene is also exacerbated by ethanol. Consequently, a narrowing of the therapeutic window for retinoids and carotenoids ensues [269].

CYP2E1, however, also, plays a useful physiologic role, and the task is now to restore a proper balance between the beneficial and the detrimental effects of the adaptive, but sometimes inappropriately excessive, CYP2E1 response to exogenous stimuli.

Acknowledgments

The skillful typing of this manuscript by Ms. Y. Rodriguez and the editorial assistance of F. DeMara are gratefully acknowledged.

References

[1] Shelmet JJ, Reichard GA, Skutches CL, et al. Ethanol causes acute inhibition of carbohydrate, fat, and protein oxidation and insulin resistance. J Clin Invest 1988;81:1137–45.

[2] Baraona E, Julkunen R, Tannenbaum L, et al. Role of intestinal bacterial overgrowth in ethanol production and metabolism in rats. Gastroenterology 1986;90:103–10.

[3] Bjorkhem I. On the role of alcohol dehydrogenase in ω-oxidation of fatty acids. Eur J Biochem 1972;30:441–51.

[4] Bosron WF, Ehrig T, Li T-K. Genetic factors in alcohol metabolism and alcoholism. Semin Liver Dis 1993;13:126–35.

[5] Parés X, Vallee BL. New human liver alcohol dehydrogenase forms with unique kinetic characteristics. Biochem Biophys Res Commun 1981;98:122–30.

[6] Moreno A, Parés X. Purification and characterization of a new alcohol dehydrogenase from human stomach. J Biochem 1991;266:1128–33.

[7] Yin S-J, Wang M-F, Liao C-S, et al. Identification of a human stomach alcohol dehydrogenase with distinctive kinetic properties. Biochem Int 1990;22:829–35.

[8] Yasunami M, Chen C-S, Yoshida A. A human alcohol dehydrogenase gene (ADH6) encoding an additional class of isozyme. Proc Natl Acad Sci USA 1991;88:7610–4.

[9] Lieber CS, DeCarli LM, Schmid R. Effects of ethanol on fatty acid metabolism in liver slices. Biochem Biophys Res Commun 1959;1:302–6.

[10] Lieber CS, Schmid R. The effect of ethanol on fatty acid metabolism: stimulation of hepatic fatty acid synthesis in vitro. J Clin Invest 1961;40:394–9.

[11] Lieber CS. Metabolism of ethanol. In: Lieber CS, editor. Medical and nutritional complications of alcoholism. New York: Plenum Medical Book Co; 1992. p. 1–35.

[12] Faller J, Fox IH. Evidence for increased urate production by activation of adenine nucleotide turnover. N Engl J Med 1982;307:1598–602.

[13] Chedid A, Mendehall CL, Gartside P, et al. Prognostic factors in alcoholic liver disease. Am J Gastroenterol 1991;82:210–6.

[14] Lane BP, Lieber CS. Ultrastructural alterations in human hepatocytes following ingestion of ethanol with adequate diets. Am J Pathol 1966;49:593–603.

[15] Lauterburg BH, Liang D, Schwarzenbach FA, et al. Mitochondrial dysfunction in alcoholic patients as assessed by breath analysis. Hepatology 1993;17:418–22.

[16] Grunnet N, Kondrup J, Dich J. Effect of ethanol on lipid metabolism in cultured hepatocytes. Biochem J 1985;228:673–81.

[17] Israel Y, Kalant H, Orrego H, et al. Experimental alcohol-induced hepatic necrosis: suppression by propylthiouracil. Proc Natl Acad Sci USA 1975;72:1137–41.

[18] Kessler BJ, Lieber JB, Bronfin GJ, et al. The hepatic blood flow and splanchnic oxygen consumption in alcohol fatty liver. J Clin Invest 1954;33:1338–45.

[19] Jauhonen P, Baraona E, Miyakawa H, et al. Mechanism for selective perivenular hepatotoxicity of ethanol. Alcohol Clin Exp Res 1982;6:350–7.

[20] Sato N, Kamada T, Kawano S, et al. Effect of acute and chronic ethanol consumption on hepatic tissue oxygen tension in rats. Pharmacol Biochem Behav 1983;18:443–7.

[21] Shaw S, Lieber CS. Increased hepatic production of alpha-amino-n-butyric acid after chronic alcohol consumption in rats and baboons. Gastroenterology 1980;78:108–13.

[22] Lieber CS, Baraona E, Hernandez-Munoz R, et al. Impaired oxygen utilization: a new mechanism for the hepatotoxicity of ethanol in sub-human primates. J Clin Invest 1989;83: 1682–90.

[23] Shaw S, Heller EA, Friedman HS, et al. Increased hepatic oxygenation following ethanol administration in baboon. Proc Soc Exp Biol Med 1977;156:509–13.

[24] Greenway CV, Lautt WW. Acute and chronic ethanol on hepatic oxygen ethanol and lactate metabolism in cats. Am J Physiol 1990;258:G411–8.

[25] Kato S, Kawase T, Alderman J, et al. Role of xanthine oxidase in ethanol-induced lipid peroxidation in rats. Gastroenterology 1990;98:203–10.

[26] Lieber CS. Alcohol and the liver: metabolism of ethanol, metabolic effects and pathogenesis of injury. Acta Med Scand Suppl 1985;703:11–55.

[27] Bond SL, Singh SM. Studies with cDNA probes on the in vivo effect of ethanol on expression of the genes of alcohol metabolism. Alcohol Alcohol 1990;25:385–94.

[28] Brighenti L, Pancaldi G. Effetto della somministrazione di alcool etilico su alcune attivita enzimatiche del fegato di ratto. Boll Soc It Biol Sper 1970;46:1–5.

[29] Lieber CS, DeCarli LM. Hepatic microsomal ethanol oxidizing system: in vitro characteristics and adaptive properties in vivo. J Biol Chem 1970;245:2505–12.

[30] Salaspuro MP, Shaw S, Jaytilleke E, et al. Attenuation of the ethanol induced hepatic redox change after chronic alcohol consumption in baboons: metabolic consequences in vivo and in vitro. Hepatology 1981;1:33–8.

[31] Ugarte G, Pino ME, Insunza I. Hepatic alcohol dehydrogenase in alcoholic addicts with and without hepatic damage. Am J Dig Dis 1967;12:589–92.

[32] Yamauchi M, Potter JJ, Mezey E. Characteristics of alcohol dehydrogenase in fat-storing (Ito) cells of rat liver. Gastroenterology 1988;94:163–9.

[33] Flisiak R, Baraona E, Li J, et al. Effects of ethanol on prostanoid production by fat-storing cells. Hepatology 1993;18:153–9.

[34] Casini A, Pellegrini G, Ceni E, et al. Human hepatic stellate cells express class I alcohol dehydrogenase and aldehyde dehydrogenase but not cytochrome P4502E1. J Hepatol 1998; 28:40–5.

[35] Day CP, Bashir R, James OF, et al. Investigation of the role of polymorphisms at the alcohol and aldehyde dehydrogenase loci in genetic predisposition to alcohol-related end-organ damage. Hepatology 1991;14:798–801.

[36] Poupon RE, Nalpas B, Coutelle C, et al. Polymorphism of alcohol dehydrogenase, alcohol and aldehyde dehydrogenase activities; implications in alcoholic cirrhosis in white patients. Hepatology 1992;15:1017–22.

[37] Lieber CS. Cytochrome P4502E1: its physiological and pathological role. Physiol Rev 1997; 77:517–44.

[38] Iseri OA, Gottlieb LS, Lieber CS. The ultrastructure of ethanol-induced fatty liver. Fed Proc 1964;23:579.

[39] Iseri OA, Lieber CS, Gottlieb LS. The ultrastructurae of fatty liver induced by prolonged ethanol ingestion. Am J Pathol 1966;48:535–55.

[40] Meldolesi J. On the significance of the hypertrophy of the smooth endoplasmic reticulum in liver cells after administration of drugs. Biochem Pharmcol 1967;16:125–31.

[41] Conney AH. Pharmacological implications of microsomal enzyme induction. Pharmacol Rev 1967;19:317–66.

[42] Lane BP, Lieber CS. Effects of butylated hydroxytoluene on the ultrastructure of rat hepatocytes. Lab Invest 1967;16:341–8.

[43] Lieber CS, DeCarli LM. Ethanol oxidation by hepatic microsomes: adaptive increase after ethanol feeding. Science 1968;162:917–8.

[44] The α-Tocopherol, β-Carotene and Cancer Prevention Study Group. The effect of vitamin E and β-carotene on the incidence of lung cancer and other cancers in male smokers. N Engl J Med 1994;330:1029–35.

[45] Teschke R, Hasumura Y, Lieber CS. Hepatic microsomal alcohol oxidizing system: solubilization, isolation and characterization. Arch Biochem Biophys 1974;163:404–15.

[46] Teschke R, Matsuzaki S, Ohnishi K, et al. Microsomal ethanol oxidizing system (MEOS): current status of its characterization and its role. Alcohol Clin Exp Res 1977;1:7–15.

[47] Ahmed S, Leo MA, Lieber CS. Interactions between alcohol and beta-carotene in patients with alcoholic liver disease. Am J Clin Nutr 1994;60:430–6.

[48] Ohnishi K, Lieber CS. Reconstitution of the microsomal ethanol-oxidizing system: qualitative and quantitative changes of cytochrome P-450 after chronic ethanol consumption. J Biol Chem 1977;252:7124–31.

[49] Miwa GT, Levin W, Thomas PE, et al. The direct oxidation of ethanol by catalase- and alcohol dehydrogenase-free reconstituted system containing cytochrome P-450. Arch Biochem Biophys 1978;187:464–75.

[50] Koop DR, Morgan ET, Tarr GE, et al. Purification and characterization of a unique isozyme of cytochrome P-450 from liver microsomes of ethanol-treated rabbits. J Biol Chem 1982; 257:8472–80.

[51] Morgan ET, Koop DR, Coon MJ. Catalytic activity of cytochrome P-450 isozyme 3a isolated from liver microsomes of ethanol-treated rabbits. J Biol Chem 1982;257:13951–7.

[52] Morgan ET, Koop DR, Coon MJ. Comparison of six rabbit liver cytochrome P-450 isozymes

in formation of a reactive metabolite of acetaminophen. Biochem Biophys Res Commun 1983;112:8–13.

[53] Ingelman-Sundberg M, Johansson I. Mechanisms of hydroxyl radical formation and ethanol oxidation by ethanol-inducible and other forms of rabbit liver microsomal cytochromes P-450. J Biol Chem 1984;259:6447–58.

[54] Yang CS, Tu YY, Koop DR, et al. Metabolism of nitrosamines by purified rabbit liver cytochrome P-450 isozymes. Cancer Res 1985;45:1140–5.

[55] Lasker JM, Raucy J, Kubota S, et al. Purification and characterization of human liver cytochrome P-450-ALC. Biochem Biophys Res Commun 1987;148:232–8.

[56] Takahashi T, Lasker JM, Rosman AS, et al. Induction of P450E1 in human liver by ethanol is due to a corresponding increase in encoding mRNA. Hepatology 1993;17:236–45.

[57] Shimizu M, Lasker JM, Tsutsumi M, et al. Immunohistochemical localization of ethanol-inducible P450IIE1 in the rat alimentary tract. Gastroenterology 1990;99:1044–53.

[58] Koivisto T, Mishin VM, Mak KM, et al. Induction of cytochrome P-4502E1 by ethanol in rat Kupffer cells. Alcohol Clin Exp Res 1996;20:207–12.

[59] Hayashi S, Watanabe J, Kaname K. Genetic polymorphism in the 5'-flanking region change transcriptional regulation of the human cytochrome P450IIE1 gene. J Biochem 1991;110: 559–65.

[60] Hirvonen A, Husgafvel-Pursiainen K, Anttila S, et al. The human CYP2E1 gene and lung cancer: Dra I and Rsa I restriction fragment length polymorphisms in a Finnish study population. Carcinogenesis 1993;14:85–8.

[61] Persson I, Johansson I, Bergling H, et al. Genetic polymorphism of cytochrome P4502E1 in a Swedish population: relation ship to incidence of lung cancer. FEBS Lett 1993;319:207–11.

[62] Uematsu F, Kikuchi H, Motomiya M, et al. Association between restriction fragment length polymorphism of the human cytochrome P450IIE1 gene and susceptibility to lung cancer. Jpn J Cancer Res 1991;82:254–6.

[63] Watanabe J, Hayashi S, Kawajiri K. Different regulations and expression of the human CYP2E1 gene due to the Rsa I polymorphism in the 5' flanking region. J Biochem 1994;116: 321–6.

[64] Tsutsumi M, Shimizu J, Lasker JM, et al. Intralobular distribution of ethanol-inducible cytochrome P-450IIE1 in liver. Hepatolgoy 1988;8:1237A.

[65] Stephens EA, Taylor JA, Kaplan N, et al. Ethnic variation in the CYP2E1 gene: polymorphism analysis of 695 African-Americans, European-Americans and Taiwanese. Pharmacogenetics 1994;4:185–92.

[66] Tsutsumi M, Takada A, Wang JS. Genetic polymorphism of cytochrome P4502E1 related to the development of alcoholic liver disease. Gastroenterology 1994;107:1430–5.

[67] Maezawa Y, Yamauchi M, Toda G. Association between restriction fragment length polymorphism of the human cytochrome P450IIE1 gene and susceptibility to alcoholic liver cirrhosis. Am J Gastroenterol 1994;89:561–5.

[68] Carr LG, Hartleroad JY, Liang YB, et al. Polymorphism at the P450IIE1 locus is not associated with alcoholic liver disease in Caucasian men. Alcohol Clin Exp Res 1995;19:182–4.

[69] Pirmohamed M, Kitteringham NR, Quest LJ, et al. Genetic polymorphism of cytochrome P4502E1 and risk of alcoholic liver disease in Caucasians. Pharmacogenetics 1995;5:351–7.

[70] Yu M-W, Gladek-Yarborough A, Santella RM, et al. Cytochrome P450 2E1 and glutathione S-transferase M1 polymorphisms and susceptibility to hepatocellular carcinoma. Gastroenterology 1995;109:1266–73.

[71] Watanabe J, Yang JP, Eguchi H, et al. An Rsa I polymorphism in the CYP2E1 gene does not affect lung cancer risk in a Japanese population. Jpn J Cancer Res 1995;86:245–8.

[72] Kato S, Shields PG, Caporaso NE, et al. Cytochrome P450IIE1 genetic polymorphisms, radical variation, and lung cancer risk. Cancer Res 1992;52:6712–5.

[73] Sugimura H, Hamada GS, Suzuki I, et al. CYP1A1 and CYP2E1 polymorphism and lung cancer, case control study in Rio de Janeiro, Brazil. Pharmacogenetics 1995;5:S145–8.

[74] Iwahashi K, Matsuo Y, Suwaki H, et al. CYP2E1 and ALDH2 genotypes and alcohol dependence in Japanese. Alcohol Clin Exp Res 1995;19:564–6.

[75] Maezawa Y, Yamauchi M, Toda G, et al. Alcohol metabolizing enzyme polymorphisms and alcoholism in Japan. Alcohol Clin Exp Res 1995;19:951–4.

[76] Kunitoh S, Tanaka T, Imaoka S, et al. Contribution of cytochrome P450s to MEOS (Microsomal Ethanol-Oxidizing System): a specific and sensitive assay of MEOS activity by HPLC with fluorescence labeling. Alcohol Alcohol 1993;28:63–8.

[77] Asai H, Imaoka S, Kuroki T, et al. Microsomal ethanol oxidizing system activity by human hepatic cytochrome P450s. J Pharmacol Exp Ther 1996;277:1004–9.

[78] Salmela KS, Kessova IG, Tsyrlov IB, et al. Respective roles of human cytochrome P4502E1, 1A2, and 3A4 in the hepatic microsomal ethanol oxidizing system. Alcohol Clin Exp Res 1998;22:2125–32.

[79] Koop DR, Tierney DJ. Multiple mechanisms in the regulation of ethanol-inducible cytochrome P-450IIE1. Bioessays 1990;9:429–35.

[80] Casazza JP, Felver ME, Veech RL. The metabolism of acetone in rat. J Biol Chem 1984; 259:231–6.

[81] Koop DR, Casazza JP. Identification of ethanol-inducible P-450 isozyme 3a as the acetone and acetol monooxygenase of rabbit microsomes. J Biol Chem 1985;260:13607–12.

[82] Reichard Jr GA, Skutches CL, Hoeldke RD, et al. Acetone metabolism in humans during diabetic ketoacidosis. Diabetes 1986;35:668–74.

[83] Casazza JP, Veech RL. The production of 1,2 propanediol in ethanol treated rats. Biochem Biophys Res Commun 1985;129:426–30.

[84] Johansson IJ, Eliasson E, Norsten C, et al. Hydroxylation of acetone by ethanol- and acetone-inducible cytochrome P450 in liver microsomes and reconstituted membranes. FEBS Lett 1986;196:59–64.

[85] Yang CS, Yoo JS, Ishizaki H, et al. Cytochrome P450IIE1: roles in nitrosamine metabolism and mechanisms of regulation. Drug Metab Rev 1990;22:147–59.

[86] Koop DR. Oxidative and reductive metabolism by cytochrome P450 2E1. FASEB J 1992;6: 724–30.

[87] Reichard Jr GA, Haff AC, Skutches CL, et al. Plasma acetone metabolism in the fasting human. J Clin Invest 1979;63:619–26.

[88] Owen OE, Trapp VE, Skutches CL, et al. Acetone metabolism during diabetic ketoacidosis. Diabetes 1982;31:242–8.

[89] Chen L, Lee M, Hong JY, et al. Relationship between cytochrome P450 2E1 and acetone catabolism in rats as studied with diallyl sulfide as an inhibitor. Biochem Pharmacol 1994;48: 2199–205.

[90] Laethem RM, Balaxy M, Falck JR, et al. Formation of 19(S)-, 19(R)- and 18(R)-hydroxyeicosatetraenoic acids by alcohol-inducible cytochrome P4502E1. J Biol Chem 1993;268: 12912–8.

[91] Amet Y, Berthou F, Goasduff T, et al. Evidence that cytochrome P450 2E1 is involved in the (ω-1)-hydroxylation of lauric acid in rat liver microsomes. Biochem Biophys Res Commun 1994;203:1168–74.

[92] Adas F, Berthou F, Picart D, et al. Involvement of cytochrome P450 2E1 in the (omega-1)-hydroxylation of oleic acid in human and rat liver microsomes. J Lipid Res 1998;39:1210–9.

[93] Ma XL, Baraona E, Lieber CS. Alcohol consumption enhances fatty acid ω-oxidation, with a greater increase in male than in female rats. Hepatology 1993;18:1247–53.

[94] Dupont I, Lucas D, Clot P, et al. Cytochrome P4502E1 inducibility and hydroxyethyl radical formation among alcoholics. J Hepatol 1998;28:564–71.

[95] Aleynik MK, Leo MA, Aleynik SI, et al. Polyenylphosphatidylcholine opposes the increase of cytochrome P4502E1 by ethanol and corrects its iron-induced decrease. Alcohol Clin Exp Res 1999;23:96–100.

[96] Aleynik MK, Lieber CS. Dilinoleoylphophatidylcholine decreases ethanol-induced cytochrome P4502E1. Biochem Biophys Res Commun 2001;288:1047–51.

[97] Lieber CS, Leo MA, Aleynik SI, et al. Polyenylphosphatidylcholine decreases alcohol-induced oxidative stress in the baboon. Alcohol Clin Exp Res 1997;21:375–9.

[98] Lieber CS, Robins S, Li J, et al. Phosphatidylcholine protects against fibrosis and cirrhosis in the baboon. Gastroenterology 1994;106:152–9.

[99] Dai Y, Rashba-Step J, Cederbaum AI. Stable expression of human cytochrome P4502E1 in HepG2 cells: characterization of catalytic activities and production of reactive oxygen intermediates. Biochemistry 1993;32:6928–37.

[100] Hetu C, Dumont A, Joly JG. Effect of chronic ethanol administration on bromobenzene liver toxicity in the rat. Toxicol Appl Pharmacol 1983;67:166–7.

[101] Siegers CP, Heidbuchel K, Younes M. Influence of alcohol, dithiocarb and (+)-catechin on the hepatotoxicity and metabolism of vinylidene chloride in rats. J Appl Toxicol 1983;3:90–5.

[102] Tsutsumi R, Leo MA, Kim C, et al. Interaction of ethanol with enflurane metabolism and toxicity: role of P450IIE1. Alcohol Clin Exp Res 1990;14:174–9.

[103] Takagi T, Alderman J, Geller J, et al. Assessment of the role of non-ADH ethanol oxidation in vivo and in hepatocytes from deermice. Biochem Pharmacol 1986;35:3601–6.

[104] Nakajima T, Okino T, Sato A. Kinetic studies on benzene metabolism in rat liver—possible presence of three forms of benzene metabolizing enzymes in the liver. Biochem Pharmacol 1987;36:2799–804.

[105] Beskid M, Bialek J, Dzieniszewski J, et al. Effect of combined phenylbutazone and ethanol administration on rat liver. Exp Pathol 1980;18:487–91.

[106] Sato C, Matsuda Y, Lieber CS. Increased hepatotoxicity of acetaminophen after chronic ethanol consumption in the rat. Gastroenterology 1981;80:140–8.

[107] Schiødt FV, Rochling FA, Casey DL, et al. Acetaminophen toxicity in an urban county hospital. N Engl J Med 1997;337:1112–7.

[108] Lieber CS, Garro A, Leo MA, et al. Alcohol and cancer. Hepatology 1986;6:1005–19.

[109] Garro AJ, Seitz HK, Lieber CS. Enhancement of dimethylnitrosamine metabolism and activation to a mutagen following chronic ethanol consumption. Cancer Res 1981;41:120–4.

[110] Seitz HK, Garro AJ, Lieber CS. Enhanced pulmonary and intestinal activation of pro-carcinogens and mutagens after chronic ethanol consumption in the rat. Eur J Clin Invest 1981; 11:33–8.

[111] Seitz HK, Czygan P, Waldherr K, et al. Ethanol and intestinal carcinogenesis in the rat. Alcohol 1985;2:491–4.

[112] Farinati F, Zhou Z, Bellah J, et al. Effect of chronic ethanol consumption on activation of nitrosopyrrolidine to a mutagen by rat upper alimentary tract, lung and hepatic tissue. Drug Metab Dispos 1985;13:210–4.

[113] Garro AJ, Lieber CS. Alcohol and cancer. Annu Rev Pharmacol Toxicol 1990;30:219–49.

[114] Nordmann R, Ribière C, Rouach H. Implication of free radical mechanisms in ethanol-induced cellular injury. Free Radic Biol Med 1992;12:219–40.

[115] DiLuzio NR. Prevention of the acute ethanol-induced fatty liver by the simultaneous administration of anti-oxidants. Life Sci 1964;3:113–9.

[116] DiLuzio NR. The role of lipid peroxidation and antioxidants in ethanol-induced lipid alterations. Exp Mol Pathol 1968;8:394–402.

[117] Castillo T, Koop DR, Kamimura S, et al. Role of cytochrome P-450 2E1 in ethanol-, carbon tetrachloride- and iron-dependent microsomal lipid peroxidation. Hepatology 1992;16:992–6.

[118] Ekstrom G, Ingelman-Sundberg M. Rat liver microsomal NADPH-supported oxidase activity and lipid peroxidation dependent on ethanol-inducible cytochrome P-450 (P-450IIE1). Biochem Pharmacol 1989;38:1313–9.

[119] Albano E, Tomasi A, Goria-Gatti L, et al. Free radical metabolism of alcohols in rat liver microsomes. Free Radic Res Commun 1987;3:243–9.

[120] Reinke L, Lai EK, DuBose CM, et al. Reactive free radical generation in vivo in heart and liver of ethanol-fed rats: correlation with radical formation in vitro. Proc Natl Acad Sci USA 1987;84:9223–7.

[121] Reinke LA, Kotake Y, McCay PB, et al. Spin trapping studies of hepatic free radicals formed following the acute administration of ethanol to rats: in vivo detection of l-hydroxyethyl radicals with PBN. Free Radic Biol Med 1991;11:31–9.

[122] Cederbaum AI. Oxygen radical generation by microsomes: role of iron and implications for alcohol metabolism and toxicity. Free Radic Biol Med 1989;7:559–67.

[123] Albano E, Tomasi A, Goria-Gatti L, et al. Role of ethanol-inducible cytochrome P-450 (P450IIE1) in catalyzing the free radical activation of aliphatic alcohols. Biochem Pharmacol 1991;411:1895–902.

[124] Clot P, Bellomo G, Tabone M, et al. Detection of antibodies against proteins modified by hydroxyethyl free radicals in patients with alcoholic cirrhosis. Gastroenterology 1995;108: 201–7.

[125] Leo MA, Lieber CS. Hepatic vitamin A depletion in alcoholic liver injury. N Engl J Med 1982;307:597–601.

[126] Sato M, Lieber CS. Hepatic vitamin A depletion after chronic ethanol consumption in baboons and rats. J Nutr 1981;111:2015–23.

[127] Leo MA, Sato M, Lieber CS. Effect of hepatic vitamin A depletion on the liver in men and rats. Gastroenterology 1983;84:562–72.

[128] Leo MA, Lowe N, Lieber CS. Interaction of drugs and retinol. Biochem Pharmacol 1986;35: 3949–53.

[129] Leo MA, Lieber CS. New pathway for retinol metabolism in liver microsomes. J Biochem 1985;260:5228–31.

[130] Leo MA, Kim CI, Lieber CS. NAD$^+$-dependent retinol dehydrogenase in liver microsomes. Arch Biochem Biophys 1987;259:241–9.

[131] Leo MA, Lieber CS. Hypervitaminosis A: a liver lover's lament. Hepatology 1988;8:412–7.

[132] Leo MA, Arai M, Sato M, et al. Hepatotoxicity of vitamin A and ethanol in the rat. Gastroenterology 1982;82:194–205.

[133] Leo MA, Lieber CS. Hepatic fibrosis after long term administration of ethanol and moderate vitamin A supplementation in the rat. Hepatology 1983;2:1–11.

[134] Heywood R, Palmer AK, Gregson RL, et al. The toxicity of beta-carotene. Toxicology 1985;36:91–100.

[135] Olson JA. Recommended dietary intakes (RDI) of vitamin A in humans. Am J Clin Nutr 1987; 45:704–16.

[136] Mobarhan S, Bowen P, Andersen B, et al. Effects of β-carotene repletion of β-carotene absorption, lipid peroxidation, and neutrophil superoxide formation in young men. Nutr Cancer 1990;14:195–206.

[137] Ward RJ, Peters TJ. The antioxidant status of patients with either alcohol-induced liver damage or myopathy. Alcohol Alcohol 1992;27:359–65.

[138] Forman MR, Beecher GR, Lanza E, et al. Effect of alcohol consumption on plasma carotenoid concentrations in premenopausal women: a controlled dietary study. Am J Clin Nutr 1995;62: 131–5.

[139] Leo MA, Kim CI, Lowe N, et al. Interaction of ethanol with β-carotene: delayed blood clearance and enhanced hepatotoxicity. Hepatology 1992;15:883–91.

[140] Leo MA, Rosman A, Lieber CS. Differential depletion of carotenoids and tocopherol in liver diseases. Hepatology 1993;17:977–86.

[141] Leo MA, Aleynik S, Aleynik M, Lieber CS. B-carotene beadlets potentiate hepatotoxicity of alcohol. Am J Clin Nutr 1997;66:1461–9.

[142] Omenn GS, Goodman GE, Thornquist MD, et al. Effects of a combination of beta carotene and vitamin A on lung cancer and cardiovascular disease. N Engl J Med 1996;334:1150–5.

[143] Leo MA, Lieber CS. Beta carotene, vitamin E, and lung cancer. N Engl J Med 1994;331:612.

[144] Albanes D, Heinonen OP, Taylor PR, et al. α-Tocopherol and β-carotene supplements and lung cancer incidence in the Alpha-Tocopherol, Beta-Carotene Cancer Prevention Study: effect of base-line characteristics and the study compliance. J Natl Cancer Inst 1996;88:1560–71.

[145] Omenn GS, Goodman GE, Thornquist MD, et al. Risk factors for lung cancer and for intervention effects in CARET, the Beta-Carotene and Retinol Efficacy Trial. J Natl Cancer Inst 1996;88:1550–9.

[146] Keilin D, Hartree EF. Properties of catalase: catalysis of coupled oxidation of alcohols. Biochem J 1945;39:293–301.

[147] Sies H, Chance B. The steady state level of catalase compound I in isolated hemoglobin-free perfused rat liver. FEBS Lett 1970;11:172–6.

[148] Handler JA, Thurman RG. Fatty acid-dependent ethanol metabolism. Biochem Biophys Res Commun 1985;133:44–51.

[149] Williamson JR, Scholz R, Browning ET, et al. Metabolic effects of ethanol in perfused rat liver. J Biol Chem 1969;25:5044–54.

[150] Handler JA, Thurman RG. Redox interactions between catalase and alcohol dehydrogenase pathways of ethanol metabolism in the perfused rat liver. J Biol Chem 1990;265:1510–5.

[151] Inatomi N, Kato S, Ito D, Lieber CS. Role of peroxisomal fatty acid beta-oxidation in ethanol metabolism. Biochem Biophys Res Commun 1989;163:418–23.

[152] Kato S, Alderman J, Lieber CS. Respective roles of the microsomal ethanol oxidizing system (MEOS) and catalase in ethanol metabolism by deermice lacking alcohol dehydrogenase. Arch Biochem Biophys 1987;254:586–91.

[153] Kato S, Alderman J, Lieber CS. Ethanol metabolism in alcohol dehydrogenase deficient deermice is mediated by the microsomal ethanol oxidizing system, not by catalase. Alcohol Alcohol 1987;1:231–4.

[154] Thurman RG, Brentzel HJ. The role of alcohol dehydrogenase in microsomal ethanol oxidation and the adaptive increase in ethanol metabolism due to chronic treatment with ethanol. Alcohol Clin Exp Res 1977;1:33–8.

[155] Lieber CS, Leo MA, Aleynik SI, et al. Polyenylphosphatidylcholine (PPC) decreases oxidant stress and protects against alcohol-induced liver injury in the baboon. Hepatology 1995; 22:225A.

[156] Kaikaus RM, Chan WK, Lysenko N, et al. Induction of liver fatty acid binding protein (l-FABP) and peroxisomal fatty acid β-oxidation by peroxisome proliferators (PP) is dependent on cytochrome p-450 activity. Hepatology 1990;12:899A.

[157] Wolff PH. Vasomotor sensitivity to alcohol in diverse mongoloid populations. Am J Hum Genet 1973;25:193–9.

[158] Goedde HW, Harada S, Agarwal DP. Racial differences in alcohol sensitivity: a new hypothesis. Hum Genet 1979;51:331–4.

[159] Harada S, Misawa S, Agarwal DP, et al. Studies on liver alcohol and acetaldehyde dehydrogenase variants in Japanese. Hoppe Seylers Z Physiol Chem 1979;360:278.

[160] Ijiri I. Studies of the relationship between the concentrations of blood acetaldehyde and urinary catecholamine and the symptoms after drinking alcohol. Jpn J Stud Alcohol 1974;9:35–9.

[161] Teng YS. Human liver aldehyde dehydrogenase in Chinese and Asiatic Indians: gene deletion and its possible implications in alcohol metabolism. Biochem Genet 1981;19:107–14.

[162] Yoshihara H, Sato N, Kamada T, et al. Low Km ALDH isozyme and alcoholic liver injury. Pharmacol Biochem Behav 1983;18:425–8.

[163] Harada S, Agarwal DP, Goedde HW, et al. Aldehyde dehydrogenase isozyme variation and alcoholism in Japan. Pharmacol Biochem Behav 1983;18:151–3.

[164] Enomoto N, Takase S, Takada N, et al. Alcoholic liver disease in heterozygotes of mutant and normal aldehyde dehydrogenase-2 genes. Hepatology 1991;13:1071–5.

[165] Hasumura Y, Teschke R, Lieber CS. Hepatic microsomal ethanol oxidizing system (MEOS): dissociation from reduced nicotinamide adenine dinucleotide phosphate-oxidase and possible role of form 1 of cytochrome P-450. J Pharmacol Exp Ther 1975;194:469–74.

[166] DiPadova C, Worner TM, Julkunen RJK, et al. Effects of fasting and chronic alcohol consumption on the first pass metabolism of ethanol. Gastroenterology 1987;92:1169–73.

[167] Espina N, Lima V, Lieber CS, et al. In vitro and in vivo inhibitory effect of ethanol and acetaldehyde on O^6-methylguanine transferase. Carcinogenesis 1988;9:761–6.

[168] Müller A, Sies H. Role of alcohol dehydrogenase activity and of acetaldehyde in ethanol-induced ethane and pentane production by isolated perfused rat liver. Biochem J 1982;206: 153–6.

[169] Müller A, Sies H. Inhibition of ethanol- and aldehyde-induced release of ethane from isolated perfused rat liver by pargyline and disulfiram. Pharmacol Biochem Behav 1983;18:429–32.

[170] Shaw S, Rubin KP, Lieber CS. Depressed hepatic glutathione and increased diene conjugates in alcoholic liver disease: evidence of lipid peroxidation. Dig Dis Sci 1983;28:585–9.

[171] Morton S, Mitchell MC. Effects of chronic ethanol feeding on glutathione turnover in the rat. Biochem Pharmacol 1985;34:1559–63.

[172] Speisky H, MacDonald A, Giles G, et al. Increased loss and decreased synthesis of hepatic glutathione after acute ethanol administration. Biochem J 1985;225:565.

[173] Hirano T, Kaplowitz N, Tsukamoto H, et al. Hepatic mitochondrial glutathione depletion and progression of experimental alcoholic liver disease in rats. Hepatology 1992;6:1423–7.

[174] Barclay LR. The cooperative antioxidant role of glutathione with a lipid-soluble and a water-soluble antioxidant during peroxidation of liposomes initiated in the aqueous phase and in the lipid phase. J Biol Chem 1988;263:16138–42.

[175] Shaw S, Jayatilleke E, Ross WA, et al. Ethanol induced lipid peroxidation: potentiation by long-term alcohol feeding and attenuation by methionine. J Lab Clin Med 1981;98:417–25.

[176] Zhang H, Loney LA, Potter BJ. Effect of chronic alcohol feeding on hepatic iron status and ferritin uptake by rat hepatocytes. Alcohol Clin Exp Res 1993;17:394–400.

[177] Valenzuela A, Fernandez V, Videla LA. Hepatic and biliary levels of flutathione and lipid peroxides following iron overload in the rat: effect of simultaneous ethanol administration. Toxicol Appl Pharmacol 1983;70:87–95.

[178] Savolainen VT, Pajarinen J, Perola M, et al. Glutathione-S-transferase GST M1 "null" genotype and the risk of alcoholic liver disease. Alcohol Clin Exp Res 1996;0:1340–5.

[179] Weiner FR, Eskreis DS, Compton KV, et al. Haplotype analysis of a type I collagen gene and its association with alcoholic cirrhosis in man. Mol Aspects Med 1988;10:159–68.

[180] Bashir R, Day CP, James FW, et al. No evidence for involvement of type I collagen structural genes in "genetic predisposition" to alcoholic cirrhosis. J Hepatol 1992;16:316–9.

[181] Geesin JC, Hendricks LJ, Falkenstein PA, et al. Regulation of collagen synthesis by ascorbic acid: characterization of the role of ascorbate-stimulated lipid peroxidation. Arch Biochem Biophys 1991;290:127–32.

[182] Tsukamoto H. Oxidative stress, antioxidants, and alcoholic liver fibrogenesis. Alcohol 1993;10:465–7.

[183] Finkelstein JD, Martin JJ. Methionine metabolism in mammals. Adaptation to methionine excess. J Biol Chem 1986;261:1582–7.

[184] Horowitz JH, Rypins EB, Henderson JM, et al. Evidence for impairment of transsulfuration pathway in cirrhosis. Gastroenterology 1981;81:668–75.

[185] Duce AM, Ortiz P, Cabrero C, et al. S-adenosyl-L-methionine synthetase and phospholipid methyltransferase are inhibited in human cirrhosis. Hepatology 1988;8:65–8.

[186] Avila MA, Carretero V, Rodriguez EN, et al. Regulation by hypoxia of methionine adenosyltrans-ferase activity and gene expression in rat hepatocytes. Gastroenterology 1998;114:364–71.

[187] Lieber CS, Casini A, DeCarli LM, et al. S-adenosyl-L-methionine attenuates alcohol-induced liver injury in the baboon. Hepatology 1990;11:165–72.

[188] Yamada S, Mak KM, Lieber CS. Chronic ethanol consumption alters rat liver plasma membranes and potentiates release of alkaline phosphatase. Gastroenterology 1985;88:1799–806.

[189] Lieber CS. Prevention and therapy with S-adenosyl-L-methionine and polyenylphosphatidyl-choline. In: Arroyo V, Bosch J, Rodes J, editors. Treatments in hepatology. Barcelona: Masson, SA; 1995. p. 299–311.

[190] Vendemiale G, Altomare E, Trizzio T, et al. Effects of oral S-adenosyl-L-methionine on hepatic glutathione in patients with liver disease. Scand J Gastroenterol 1989;24:407–15.

[191] Mato JM, Cámara J, Fernández de Paz J, et al. S-Adenosylmethionine in alcoholic liver cirrhosis: a randomized, placebo-controlled, double-blind, multicentre clinical trial. J Hepatol 1999;30:1081–9.

[192] Halliwell B, Gutteridge JMC. Lipid peroxidation: a radical chain reaction. In: Halliwell B, Gutteridge JMC, editors. Free radicals in biology and medicine. 2nd edition. Oxford: Clarendon Press; 1989. p. 188–276.

[193] Aleynik SI, Leo MA, Ma X, et al. Polyenylphosphatidylcholine (PPC) prevents carbon tetrachloride-induced lipid peroxidation while it attenuates liver fibrosis. J Hepatol 1997;27: 554–61.

[194] Lieber CS. Role of oxidative stress and antioxidant therapy in alcoholic and non-alcoholic liver diseases. In: Sies H, editor. Advances in pharmacology, Vol. 38. San Diego (CA): Academic Press; 1997. p. 601–28.

[195] Arai M, Gordon ER, Lieber CS. Decreased cytochrome oxidase activity in hepatic mitochondria after chronic ethanol consumption and the possible role of decreased cytochrome aa_3 content and changes in phospholipids. Biochim Biophys Acta 1984;797:320–7.

[196] Lieber CS, Robins SJ, Leo MA. Hepatic phosphatidylethanolamine methyltransferase activity is decreased by ethanol and increased by phosphatidylcholine. Alcohol Clin Exp Res 1994; 18:592–5.

[197] Lieber CS, Li JI, Robins S, DeCarli LM, Mak KM, Leo MA. Dietary dilinoleoylphosphatidyl-choline (DLPC) is incorporated into liver phospholipids, protects against alcoholic cirrhosis, enhances collagenase activity and prevents acetaldehyde-induced collagen accumulation in cultured lipocytes. Hepatology 1992;16:87A.

[198] Fox JM. Polyene phosphatidylcholine: pharmacokinetics after oral administrationa review. In: Avogaro P, Macini M, Ricci G, Paoletti R, editors. Phospholipids and atherosclerosis. New York: Raven Press; 1983. p. 65–80.

[199] Li J-J, Kim C-I, Leo MA, et al. Polyunsaturated lecithin prevents acetaldehyde-mediated hepatic collagen accumulation by stimulating collagenase activity in cultured lipocytes. Hepatology 1992;15:373–81.

[200] Ma X, Zhao J, Lieber CS. Polyenylphosphatidylcholine attenuates non-alcoholic hepatitis fibrosis and accelerates its regression. J Hepatol 1996;24:604–13.

[201] Navder KP, Baraona E, Lieber CS. Effects of polyenylphosphatidylcholine (PPC) on alcohol-induced fatty liver and hyperlipemia in rats. J Nutr 1996;127:1800–6.

[202] Bjørneboe GEA, Bjørneboe A, Hagen BF, et al. Reduced hepatic α-tocopherol content after long-term administration of ethanol to rats. Biochem Biophys Acta 1987;918:236–41.

[203] Kawase T, Kato S, Lieber CS. Lipid peroxidation and antioxidant defense systems in rat liver after chronic ethanol feeding. Hepatology 1989;10:815–21.

[204] Leo MA, Rosman AS, Lieber CS. Differential depletion of carotenoids and tocopherol in liver disease. Hepatology 1993;17:977–86.

[205] von Herbay A, de Groot H, Hegi U, et al. Low vitamin E content in plasma of patients with alcoholic liver disease, hemochromatosis and Wilson's disease. J Hepatol 1994;20:41–6.

[206] Seitz HK, Poschl G. Antioxidant drugs and colchicine in the treatment of alcoholic liver disease. In: Arroyo V, Bosch J, Rodes J, editors. Treatments in hepatology. Barcelona: Masson, S.A.; 1995. p. 271–6.

[207] Cortot A, Jobin G, Fucrot F, et al. Gastric emptying and gastrointestinal absorption of al-cohol ingested with a meal. Dig Dis Sci 1986;31:343–8.

[208] Julkunen RJK, DiPadova C, Lieber CS. First pass metabolism of ethanol: a gastrointestinal barrier against the systemic toxicity of ethanol. Life Sci 1985;37:567–73.

[209] Julkunen RJK, Tannenbaum L, Baraona E, et al. First pass metabolism of ethanol: an impor-tant determinant of blood levels after alcohol consumption. Alcohol 1985;2:437–41.

[210] Pestalozzi DM, Buhler R, von Wartburg JP, et al. Immunohistochemical localization of al-cohol dehydrogenase in the human gastrointestinal tract. Gastroenteroloy 1983;85:1011–6.

[211] Hernández-Muñoz R, Caballeria J, Baraona E, et al. Human gastric alcohol dehydrogenase: its inhibition by H_2-receptor antagonists, and its effect on the bioavailability of ethanol. Alcohol Clin Exp Res 1990;14:946–50.

[212] Stone CL, Thomason HR, Bosron WF, et al. Purification and partial amino acid sequence of a high activity human stomach alcohol dehydrogenase. Alcohol Clin Exp Res 1993;17:911–8.

[213] Farrés J, Moreno A, Crosas B, et al. Alcohol dehydrogenase of class IV (δADH) from human stomach; cDNA sequence and structure/function relationships. Eur J Biochem 1994; 224:549–57.

[214] Yokoyama H, Baraona E, Lieber CS. Molecular cloning of human class IV alcohol dehydrogenase. Biochem Biophys Res Commun 1994;203:219–24.

[215] Satre MA, Zgombic-Knight M, Duester G. The complete structure of human class IV alcohol dehydrogenase (Retinol Dehydrogenase) determined from ADH7 Gene. J Biol Chem 1994;269: 15606–12.

[216] Yokoyama H, Baraona E, Lieber CS. Molecular cloning and chromosomal localization of ADH7 gene encoding human class IV ADH. Genomics 1996;31:243–5.

[217] Yokoyama H, Baraona E, Lieber CS. Upstream structure of human ADH7 gene and the organ distribution of its expression. Biochem Biophys Res Commun 1995;216:216–22.

[218] Mirmiran-Yazdy SA, Haber PS, Korsten MA, et al. Metabolism of ethanol in rat gastric cells and its inhibition by cimetidine. Gastroenterology 1995;108:737–42.

[219] Haber PS, Gentry T, Mak KM, et al. Metabolism of alcohol by human gastric cells: relation to first pass metabolism. Gastroenterology 1996;111:863–70.

[220] Levitt MD, Levitt DG. The critical role of the rate of ethanol absorption in the interpretation of studies purporting to demonstrate gastric metabolism of ethanol. J Pharmacol Exp Ther 1994;269:297–304.

[221] Lieber CS, Gentry RT, Baraona E. First pass metabolism of ethanol. In: Saunders JB, Whitfield JB, editors. The biology of alcohol problems. UK: Elsevier Science Publishers; 1996. p. 315–26.

[222] Smith T, DeMaster EG, Furne JK, et al. First-pass gastric mucosal metabolism of ethanol is negligible in the rat. J Clin Invest 1992;89:1801–6.

[223] Sato N, Kitamura T. First-pass metabolism of ethanol: an overview. Gastroenterology 1996; 111:1143–4.

[224] Lim Jr RT, Gentry RT, Ito D, et al. First pass metabolism of ethanol in rats is predominantly gastric. Alcohol Clin Exp Res 1993;17:1337–44.

[225] Roine RP, Gentry RT, Hernández-Muñoz R, et al. Aspirin increases blood alcohol concentrations in human after ingestion of ethanol. JAMA 1990;264:2406–8.

[226] Caballeria J, Baraona E, Rodamilans M, et al. Effects of cimetidine on gastric alcohol dehydrogenase activity and blood ethanol levels. Gastroenterology 1989;96:388–92.

[227] Stone CL, Hurley TD, Peggs CF, et al. Cimetidine inhibition of human gastric and liver alcohol dehydrogenase isoenzymes: identification of inhibitor complexes by kinetics and molecular modeling. Biochemistry 1995;34:4008–14.

[228] Amir I, Anwar N, Baraona E, et al. Ranitidine increases the bioavailability of imbibed alcohol by accelerating gastric emptying. Life Sci 1996;58:511–8.

[229] Fraser AG, Hudson M, Sawyer AM, et al. Short report: the effect of ranitidine on postprandial absorption of a low dose of alcohol. Aliment Pharmacol Ther 1992;6:267–71.

[230] Palmer RH, Frank WO, Nambi P, et al. Effects of various concomitant medications on gastric alcohol dehydrogenase and first-pass metabolism of ethanol. Am J Gastrol 1991;86:1749–55.

[231] Gupta AM, Baraona E, Lieber CS. Significant increase of blood alcohol by cimetidine after repetitive drinking of small alcohol doses. Alcohol Clin Exp Res 1995;19:1083–7.

[232] Klein KE, Breuker K, Brüner H, et al. Blutalkohol und Fluguntuchtigkeit. Versuch einer Erarbeitung von Richtwerten für die allgemeine Luftfahrt. Int Z Angew Physiol 1967;24: 254–7.

[233] Modell JG, Mountz JM. Drinking and flying—the problem of alcohol use in pilots. N Engl J Med 1990;323:455–61.

[234] Moskowitz H, Burns MM, Williams AF. Skill performance at low blood alcohol levels. J Stud Alcohol 1985;46:482–5.

[235] Baraona E, Yokoyama A, Ishii H, et al. Lack of alcohol dehydrogenase isoenzyme activities in the stomach of Japanese subjects. Life Sci 1991;49:1929–34.

[236] Dohmen K, Baraona E, Ishibadsshi H, et al. Ethnic differences in gastric sigma alcohol dehydrogenase activity and ethanol first pass metabolism. Alcohol Clin Exp Res 1996;20: 1569–76.

[237] Battiston L, Moretti M, Tulissi P, et al. Hepatic glutathione determination after ethanol administration in rat: evidence of the first-pass metabolism of ethanol. Life Sci 1995;56:241–8.

[238] Iimuro Y, Bradford BU, Forman DT, et al. Glycine prevents alcohol-induced liver injury by decreasing alcohol in the rat stomach. Gastroenterology 1996;110:1536–42.

[239] Becker U, Deis A, Sorenson TIA, et al. Prediction of risk of liver disease by alcohol intake, sex, and age: a prospective population study. Hepatology 1996;23:1025–9.

[240] Morgan MY, Sherlock S. Sex-related differences among 100 patients with alcoholic liver disease. BMJ 1977;1:939–41.

[241] Parrish KM, Dufour MC, Stinson FS, et al. Average daily alcohol consumption during adult life among decedents with and without cirrhosis: The 1986 National Mortality Followback Survey. J Stud Alcohol 1993;54:450–6.

[242] Pequignot G, Tuyns AJ, Berta JL. Ascitic cirrhosis in relation to alcohol consumption. Int J Epidemiol 1978;7:113–20.

[243] Mann K, Batra A, Günthner A, et al. Do women develop alcoholic brain damage more readily than men? Alcohol Clin Exp Res 1992;16:1052–6.

[244] Frezza M, Di Padova C, Pozzato G, et al. High blood alcohol levels in women. The role of decreased gastric alcohol dehydrogenase activity and first-pass metabolism. N Engl J Med 1990;322:95–9.

[245] Seitz HK, Egerer G, Simanowski UA, et al. Human gastric alcohol dehydrogenase activity: effect of age, gender and alcoholism. Gut 1993;34:1433–7.

[246] Roine RP, Gentry RT, Lim Jr RT, et al. Effect of concentration of ingested ethanol on blood alcohol levels. Alcohol Clin Exp Res 1991;15:734–8.

[247] Roine RP, Gentry RT, Lim Jr RT, et al. Comparison of blood alcohol concentrations after beer and whiskey. Alcohol Clin Exp Res 1993;17:709–11.

[248] Pateron D, Fabre M, Ink O, et al. Influence de l'alcool et de la cirrhose sur la présence de Helicobacter pylori dans la muqueuse gastrique. Gastroenterol Clin Biol 1990;14:555–60.

[249] Nagy L, Kusstatscher S, Hauschka PV, et al. Role of cysteine proteases and protease inhibitors in gastric mucosal damage induced by ethanol or ammonia in the rat. J Clin Invest 1996;98: 1047–54.

[250] Lieber CS. Gastric ethanol metabolism and gastritis: interactions with other drugs, helicobacter pylori, and antibiotic therapy (1957–1997)—a review. Alcohol Clin Exp Res 1997;21:1360–6.

[251] Lieber CS, Lefevre A. Effect of oxytetracycline on acidity, ammonia and urea in gastric juice in normal and uremic subjects. C R Soc Biol (Paris) 1957;151:1038–42.

[252] Meyers S, Lieber CS. Reduction of gastric ammonia by ampicillin in normal and azotemic subjects. Gastroenterology 1976;70:244–7.

[253] Uppal R, Lateef SK, Korsten MA, et al. Chronic alcoholic gastritis: roles of ethanol and helicobacter pylori. Arch Intern Med 1991;151:760–4.

[254] Wickramasinghe SN, Gardner B, Barden G. Circulating cytotoxic protein generated after ethanol consumption: identification and mechanism of reaction with cells. Lancet 1987;2: 122–6.

[255] Sohda T, Mizuno K, Momose Y, et al. Studies on antidiabetic agents. 11. Novel thiazolidinedione derivatives as potent hypoglycemic and hypolipidemic agents. J Med Chem 1992;35:2617–26.

[256] Norton ID, Apte MV, Dixson H, et al. Cystic fibrosis genotypes and alcoholic pancreatitis. J Gastroenterol Hepatol 1998;13:496–9.

[257] Kessova IG, DeCarli LM, Lieber CS. Inducibility of cytochromes P4502E1 & P4501A1 in rat pancreas. Alcohol Clin Exp Res 1998;22:501–4.

[258] Ding X, Koop DR, Crump BL, et al. Immunochemical identification of cytochrome P-450 isozyme 3a (P-450ALC) in rabbit nasal and kidney microsomes and evidence for differential induction by alcohol. Mol Pharmacol 1986;30:370–6.

[259] Ding X, Coon MJ. Purification and characterization of two unique forms of cytochrome P-450 from rabbit nasal microsomes. Biochemistry 1988;27:8330–7.

[260] Lieber CS. Microsomal ethanol-oxidizing system (MEOS), the first 30 years (1968–1998)— a review. Alcohol Clin Exp Res 1999;23:991–1007.

[261] Raucy JL, Lasker JM, Kraner JC, et al. Induction of P450IIE1 in the obese rat. Mol Pharmacol 1991;39:275–80.

[262] Weltman MD, Farrell GC, Hall P, et al. Hepatic cytochrome P4502E1 is increased in patients with nonalcoholic steatohepatitis. Hepatology 1998;27:128–33.

[263] Lieber CS, Leo MA, Mak KM, et al. Model of non-alcoholic steatohepatitis. Am J Clin Nutr 2004;79:502–9.

[264] James FW, Day CP. Non-alcoholic steatohepatitis (NASH): a disease of emerging identity and importance. J Hepatol 1998;29:495–501.

[265] Yu AS, Keeffe EB. Nonalcoholic fatty liver disease. Rev Gastroenterol Disord 2002;2:11–9.

[266] Mogelson S, Lange LG. Nonoxidative ethanol metabolism in rabbit myocardium: purification to homogeneity of fatty acyl ethyl ester synthase. Biochemistry 1984;23:4075–81.

[267] Laposata EA, Lange LG. Presence of nonoxidative ethanol metabolism in human organs commonly damaged by ethanol abuse. Science 1986;231:497–9.

[268] Werner J, Laposata M, Fernandez-Del Castillo C, et al. Pancreatic injury in rats induced by fatty acid ethyl ester, a nonoxidative metabolite of alcohol. Gastroenterology 1997;113:286–94.

[269] Leo MA, Lieber CS. Alcohol, vitamin A, and beta-carotene: adverse interactions, including hepatotoxicity and cacinogencity. Am J Clin Nutr 1999;69:1071–85.

ELSEVIER
SAUNDERS

Clin Liver Dis 9 (2005) 37–53

CLINICS IN
LIVER DISEASE

Morphology of Alcoholic Liver Disease

Jay H. Lefkowitch, MD

*Columbia University, Department of Surgical Pathology, PH 1564W, 630 W 168th Streest,
VC 14th Floor, Room 215, New York, NY 10032, USA*

Since Mallory's seminal description of the pathology of alcoholic hepatitis [1], the morphology of alcoholic liver injury has been described in many original investigations and in reviews [2–5]. More recently, exceptional interest in hepatic stellate cells [6] and studies addressing the problem of hepatic steatosis [7–11] have expanded the perspective on the mechanisms of cellular injury and fibrosis due to alcohol. Attention to the fatty liver has grown as obesity and diabetes have become increasingly prevalent, contributing to numerous studies concerning nonalcoholic fatty liver disease (NAFLD) [12], which are also relevant to alcoholic liver injury. Indeed, alcoholic disease and NAFLD share many morphologic and pathogenetic features. In both conditions important roles are played by tumor necrosis factor-α [10], stellate cell activation [11], and formation of protein adducts [13], topics that are covered elsewhere in this issue. This paper reviews the morphologic features of alcoholic liver disease (ALD) (Box 1).

Steatosis

The first and most predictable hepatic change attributable to alcohol is development of large droplet (macrovesicular) steatosis (fatty change, fatty liver). This characteristically is most prominent in centrilobular regions (Fig. 1), but in more severe cases may involve the entire lobule. Lipid vacuoles occupy much of the hepatocyte cytoplasm, pushing the nucleus and other organelles to the periphery of the cell (Fig. 2). The lipid vacuoles comprise triglycerides, fatty acids, monoglycerides, and diglycerides [14]. The presence of intracellular fat is a stimulus for lipid peroxidation and generation of lipid peroxidation byproducts

E-mail address: jhl3@columbia.edu

Box 1. Major pathologic lesions in alcoholic liver disease

- **Steatosis**
    Large droplet (macrovesicular)
    Small droplet (microvesicular):
        Alcoholic foamy degeneration
- **Alcoholic steatohepatitis (ASH)**
- **Cirrhosis**
- **Other associated conditions**
    Hepatitis B and C
    Iron overload
    Biliary obstruction (eg, pancreatitis)
    Hepatocellular carcinoma

---

such as malondialdehyde [13]. The importance of lipid peroxidation as one of several factors involved in the pathogenesis of steatohepatitis has been recognized recently [15], particularly in studies of individuals with NAFLD.

Hepatocyte death by apoptosis occurs in the alcoholic fatty liver [16] (particularly in alcoholic steatohepatitis), and has been demonstrated in rats and mice after ethanol feeding [17]. Factors involved in precipitating apoptosis in this setting appear to include tumor necrosis factor-α and expression of Fas on the surface of hepatocytes [16]. Activation of this pathway of cell death in fatty liver reduces functional liver-cell mass, and may in turn incite necrosis and macrophage phagocytic activity [16]. Although extensive hepatocyte apoptosis in the

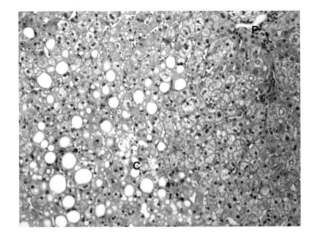

Fig. 1. Centrilobular large droplet steatosis. Hepatocytes in the centrilobular region (C) contain large droplet fat. Hepatocytes near the portal tract (P) are spared. Hematoxylin and eosin stain.

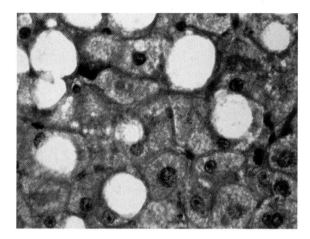

Fig. 2. Macrovesicular steatosis. Large lipid vacuoles within hepatocytes occupy the majority of the cytoplasm, pushing the nucleus to the periphery of the cell. Hematoxylin and eosin stain.

fatty liver is unusual (eg, in comparison to chronic hepatitis C), discrete apoptotic bodies may be found on careful examination of tissue sections (Fig. 3).

A minor component of the alcoholic fatty liver may be small droplet (microvesicular) steatosis. However, an uncommon form of ALD (alcoholic foamy degeneration [18]) shows a predominance of small droplet fat, usually accentuated in perivenular regions (Fig. 4). This condition was first reported by Uchida and colleagues [18] in patients with chronic alcohol ingestion and acute hepatic decompensation, but without associated inflammation or progression to fibrosis. Liver function tests, particularly gamma glutamyl transferase activity, may be substantially higher than in typical alcoholic steatohepatitis [19].

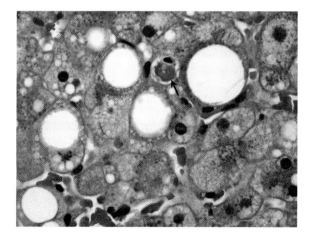

Fig. 3. Apoptosis in fatty liver. One apoptotic body (*arrow*) is seen in within a sinusoidal space. The liver is mildly fatty. Hematoxylin and eosin stain.

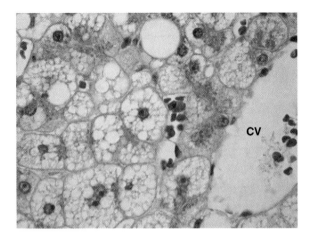

Fig. 4. Alcoholic foamy degeneration. This unusual type of alcoholic liver disease shows a predominance of microvesicular (small droplet) fat in hepatocytes. Note that the hepatocyte nuclei remain in a central or near-central position within the cell, in contrast to large droplet fat. CV, centrilobular vein. Hematoxylin and eosin stain.

Macrovesicular steatosis in ALD may be associated with scattered small collections of lymphocytes in the lobules (Fig. 5) . This type of minor inflammation in alcoholic fatty liver can be considered analogous to a similar lesion in nonalcoholics that has been designated as NAFLD type 2 [20]. Rupture of hepatocellular fat may also result in lipogranuloma formation [21]. Hepatocytes may contain megamitochondria [22], visible on hematoxylin and eosin-stained sections as ovoid or rounded eosinophilic cytoplasmic inclusions measuring between 2 to 10 μm across (Fig. 6). Megamitochondria are also seen in NAFLD

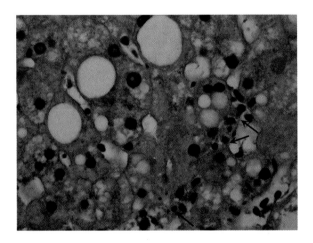

Fig. 5. Focal inflammation in alcoholic fatty liver. A few clusters of lobular lymphocytes (*arrows*) are often seen in otherwise simple fatty liver due to alcohol use. Hematoxylin and eosin stain.

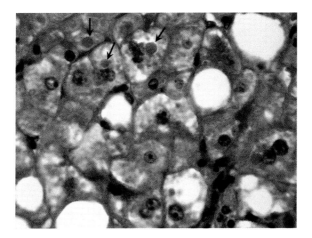

Fig. 6. Megamitochondria in alcoholic liver disease. The round, eosinophilic inclusions within hepatocytes (*arrows*) are giant mitochondria. They may be seen in both steatosis and steatohepatitis. Hematoxylin and eosin stain.

[23], and are therefore not specific for alcoholic liver injury. They may also be evident in steatohepatitis [24].

Steatohepatitis

The histopathologic changes that constitute steatohepatitis have been well described in both alcoholics [3] and nonalcoholics [25], for which the terms alcoholic steatohepatitis (ASH) and nonalcoholic steatohepatitis (NASH) are

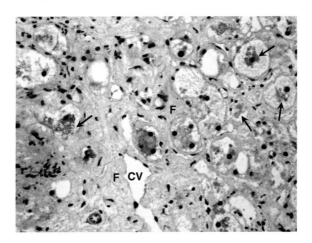

Fig. 7. Alcoholic steatohepatitis. Marked steatohepatitis is evident around the centrilobular vein (CV). Hepatocytes are ballooned and many contain Mallory bodies (*arrows*). Extensive pericellular fibrosis is present (F). In this example, only minimal fat is seen. Hematoxylin and eosin stain.

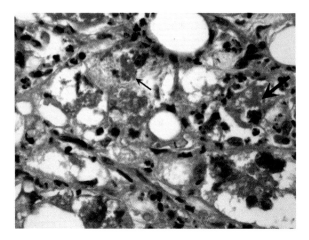

Fig. 8. Alcoholic steatohepatitis. Hepatocytes show marked hydropic ballooning (particularly prominent at lower right corner) and intracytoplasmic Mallory bodies (*arrows*). Note the neutrophil satellitosis around hepatocytes with Mallory bodies. Hematoxylin and eosin stain.

used, respectively. The broad picture of steatohepatitis affects perivenular regions in its earliest stage and includes the presence of hepatocellular damage, inflammation and, importantly, fibrosis. The full constellation of histopathologic findings includes steatosis, hepatocellular ballooning with cytoplasmic rarefaction, inflammation with neutrophils or lymphocytes, intracytoplasmic Mallory bodies in hepatocytes, and fibrosis with a perivenular, perisinusoidal, and pericellular disposition (Figs. 7–9). Affected hepatocytes in steatohepatitis appear bloated, with a wispy, rarefied cytoplasm (Figs. 7 and 8). Mallory bodies (alcoholic hyalin) (Figs. 7–9) appear as rope-like strands, clumps, or aggregates

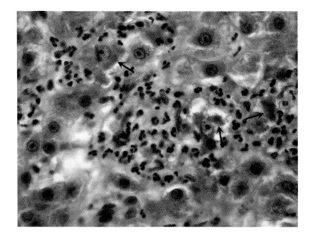

Fig. 9. Alcoholic steatohepatitis. In this example there is a marked neutrophil infiltrate and little fat. Mallory bodies are also present (*arrows*). Hematoxylin and eosin stain.

of eosinophilic material within the cytoplasm of hepatocytes (often near or surrounding the nucleus). Hepatocyte death may result in their extrusion into the extracellular space. Their chief components are cytoskeletal intermediate filaments, endowing them with positive immunostaining for cytokeratins 8 and 18 [4,26,27]. The Mallory body has been considered a "sequestosome" [28], a product of cellular stress, whose constituents include not only polyphosphory-lated intermediate filament-type cytokeratins, but also p62 (a phosphotyrosine-independent ligand in the family of cytoplasmic kinases [29]) and ubiquitin (cellular chaperone for proteins fated for degradation). Immunohistochemical staining for ubiquitin is thereby useful in corroborating the presence of Mallory bodies (Fig. 10). This can be particularly helpful in diagnosing milder forms of steatohepatitis in which there is only minimal hepatocyte ballooning and little or no fat.

Inflammation in ASH is typically neutrophil-rich, with "satellitosis" around or even into hepatocytes containing Mallory bodies (Fig. 9). Lymphocytes may also be present, or the predominant inflammatory cells in some cases. Activated Kupffer cells, some of which contain lipid vacuoles, are also in the background inflammatory infiltrate of steatohepatitis [30], although they are relatively inapparent on routine microscopy.

The perivenular and perisinusoidal fibrosis of steatohepatitis is an important and distinctive feature resulting from activation of stellate cells (Figs. 7 and 11). Collagen stains, including trichrome and reticulin methods, highlight the "chicken-wire" pattern of fibrosis in centrilobular regions (Fig. 12). More severe cases may be associated with venous occlusion [31]. In typical steato-hepatitis there is thickening of the walls of central veins with tendrils of fibrosis extending beyond into the perisinusoidal spaces and surrounding hepatocytes (Fig. 11). The adjacent parenchyma displays the changes described above, or

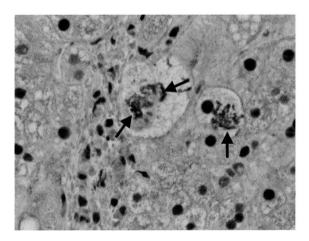

Fig. 10. Ubiquitin in Mallory bodies. Brown reaction product marks the ubiquitin within Mallory body material present in these hepatocytes. Specific immunoperoxidase for ubiquitin.

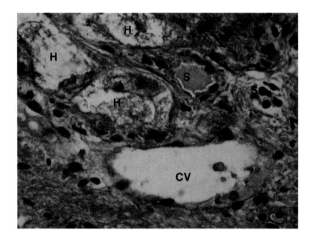

Fig. 11. Perivenular and pericellular fibrosis in alcoholic steatohepatitis. An extensive network of fibrosis (stained blue) surrounds the central vein (CV) and infiltrates the perisinusoidal spaces. S, sinusoid, H, hepatocyte. Masson trichrome stain.

if the steatohepatitis is quiescent, there will be little cellular damage or inflammation. The distribution (ie, perivenular) and appearance of the fibrosis in the latter instance presents a fairly limited differential diagnosis including various forms of hepatic venous outflow obstruction (including chronic cardiac failure), hypervitaminosis A [32], and diabetes [33].

The portal tracts appear relatively normal in early steatohepatitis that is confined to centrilobular regions. Mild portal lymphocytic infiltrates may be present in some alcoholics [34]. If generalized, such infiltrates should raise consideration of concomitant chronic hepatitis (see Other conditions associated

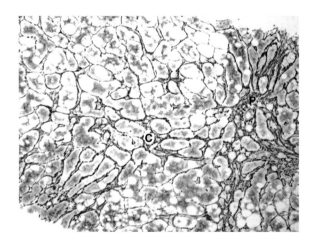

Fig. 12. "Chicken-wire" perivenular fibrosis in alcoholic steatohepatitis. This characteristic pattern of fibrosis in centrilobular regions (C) is highlighted by reticulin stain. P, portal tract. Reticulin stain.

with alcoholic liver disease). Significant portal tract changes develop, however, when perivenular steatohepatitis extends sufficiently far into the periphery of lobules as to reach the portal tracts, as discussed below.

Progression of steatohepatitis to cirrhosis

The perivenular fibrosis of ASH has been cited as an important predictor of progression to cirrhosis unless alcohol exposure is abated [35]. Morphologic progression may proceed by two major routes: one characterized by fibrosis, which bridges between central veins (Fig. 13), and the second by fibrosis linking central veins to portal tracts (Fig. 14). The latter route perhaps constitutes the more serious of the two from the vantage point of altered liver synthetic and metabolic function. Formation of vascularized fibrous septa between central veins and portal tracts is likely to result in portal-to-central vascular shunting with considerable hepatic blood flow bypassing parenchymal clearance. From a morphologic standpoint, the engagement of portal tracts in the inflammatory and fibrosing process of steatohepatitis is an important trigger of a ductular reaction (bile ductular proliferation) (Fig. 14), which may evolve alongside and within the developing bridges of fibrosis. The newly formed ductular structures, probably derived from progenitor cells present in the affected regions, often obscure the original sites of portal tracts by migration along the paths of bridging fibrous septa. The portal tracts become secondarily inflamed (neutrophils and lymphocytes) and fibrotic because of the encroachment of steatohepatitis. Because liver biopsy material viewed down the microscope represents a two-dimensional view of this process, the various planes in which a given biopsy sample is cut may influence how this progressive steatohepatitic lesion appears. For example,

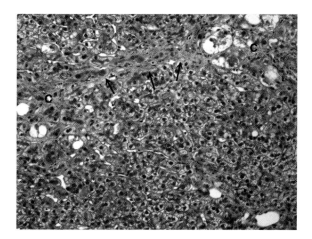

Fig. 13. Central-to-central bridging fibrosis in progressive steatohepatitis. A bridge of fibrosis (*arrows*) links two centrilobular regions (C). Masson trichrome stain.

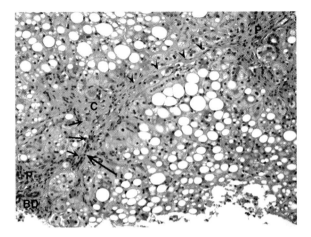

Fig. 14. Central-to-portal bridging fibrosis in progressive steatohepatitis. A centrilobular region is being linked to two portal tracts (P) by bridging fibrosis (*arrows and arrowheads*). In the portal tract at the lower left there is a native bile duct (BD) as well as a reactive ductular structure (*long arrow*) migrating along the fibrous septum toward the centrilobular region (C). Hematoxylin and eosin stain.

there may be seemingly isolated inflamed portal tracts with irregular periportal fibrosis and a ductular reaction, suggesting that a separate portal tract pathology is present. Yet such tracts are likely to be linked to perivenular areas of steatohepatitis that are present in another tissue plane not seen in the section. The corollary of this point is that isolated portal tract pathology should be a signal to the pathologist for close examination of perivenular regions for the changes of steatohepatitis. Portal tract inflammation with fibrosis or ductular reaction in the

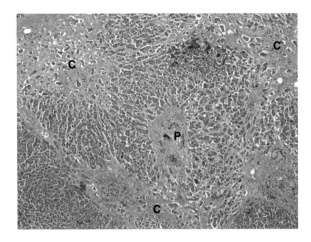

Fig. 15. Reversed lobulation in late alcoholic liver disease. The relatively normal portal tract (P) appears as if at the center of a lobule of parenchyma, the periphery consisting of the extensively scarred centrilobular (C) regions. Hematoxylin and eosin stain.

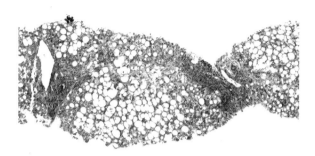

Fig. 16. Developing cirrhosis. This needle biopsy with marked steatosis has a nodular contour due to developing cirrhosis. Hematoxylin and eosin stain.

absence of steatohepatitis otherwise may reflect the presence of chronic hepatitis or biliary tract disease (see Other lesions in alcoholic liver disease). On the other hand, some portal tracts may remain unengaged by steatohepatitis and will appear normal or close to normal. This results in the appearance of "reversed lobulation" (Fig. 15), in which normal portal tracts come to appear as the centers of parenchymal units, with the scarred perivenular regions now appearing to be at the periphery of surviving parenchyma.

In the progressive stage of steatohepatitis with extensive bridging fibrosis, the net result is the subdivision of the liver parenchyma into units the size of lobules

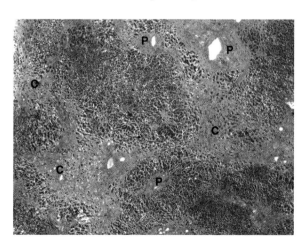

Fig. 17. Poststeatohepatitic fibrosis without regeneration. There has been prior steatohepatitis affecting centrilobular regions (C), with resultant perivenular, perisinusoidal, and pericellular fibrosis. Bridging fibrosis interconnects central veins to portal tracts (P) and nearly obliterates some lobules. Note the absence of significant regenerative nodule formation. Masson trichrome stain.

or smaller by fibrosis, the future "micronodular cirrhosis" (Fig. 16). However, there is often greater fibrosis than there is hepatocellular regeneration, with resultant isolation of remaining cords or clusters of hepatocytes within fibrous tissue (Fig. 17). This lack of regeneration may explain the high short-term mortality of approximately 50% in those with severe steatohepatitis [36]. There may be continued evidence of hepatocellular damage, fat, and inflammation in the surviving parenchyma. Cholestasis, not usually a major feature of simple perivenular steatohepatitis, is often prominent because of interrupted bile flow by fibrosis. Broad areas of replacement fibrosis may obliterate contiguous lobules, and are frequently evident macroscopically in explanted livers or at post-mortem examination. Evolution to macronodules or a macronodular cirrhosis may occur with prolonged abstinence. Hepatocellular carcinoma develops in some 5% to 15% of patients with ALD [5], often in the setting of macronodular cirrhosis [5]. Concomitant risk factors such as chronic hepatitis C and iron overload may contribute to the risk of carcinoma.

Grading and staging of steatohepatitis

Grading of necroinflammatory activity and staging of fibrosis are now actively used in assessment of chronic hepatitis [37–40]. For ASH, however, no formal system has been adopted by consensus, but the scoring procedure for NASH described by Brunt and colleagues [41] could be readily adapted for use in ASH. The basic premise of such a scoring system delineates the extent of involvement of lobular parenchyma by hepatocellular damage and inflammation as grades 1, 2, and 3, while the degree of fibrosis is categorized from stage 1 to stage 4 (cirrhosis).

Other conditions associated with alcoholic liver disease

The histopathology of ALD may be modified by coexisting conditions, particularly chronic viral hepatitis, large bile duct obstruction due to pancreatitis, and iron overload, which are prevalent in this patient population. Antibodies to hepatitis C virus (HCV) are found in as many as 35% to 40% of alcoholics [42,43], and chronic HCV infection increases the severity of liver disease [44]. The presence of portal tract lymphoid aggregates or follicles and periportal interface hepatitis microscopically should prompt investigation of HCV serology if this has not previously been obtained. Although serologic evidence of prior hepatitis B virus infection is common in alcoholics, this does not appear to affect disease severity [43,44].

Morphologic features of biliary tract disease may be present if there is either acute or chronic pancreatitis due to alcohol. As indicated earlier, significant cholestasis is not usually seen in association with either macrovesicular steatosis or early perivenular steatohepatitis, but it may become prominent when

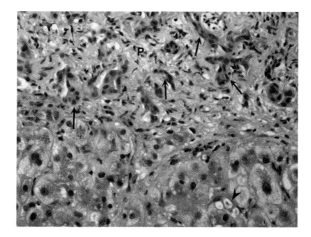

Fig. 18. Pancreatitis with chronic large bile duct obstruction. The portal tract (P) shows changes of chronic biliary obstruction, including mild edema, portal and periportal fibrosis, and a prominent ductular reaction (*arrows*). A mild infiltrate of lymphocytes and neutrophils is also present. Cholestasis (*arrowhead*) at the lobular periphery reflects the chronicity of this process and the direct obstructive effects of portal and periportal fibrosis. Hematoxylin and eosin stain.

pancreatitis is present. The accompanying portal tract changes include edema, neutrophil infiltrate, and ductular reaction. With chronic pancreatitis there may be superimposed portal and periportal fibrosis [45] (Fig. 18).

Hepatic iron overload is common in ALD. This is most often secondary iron overload due to a number of possible factors including increased intestinal iron absorption, prior transfusion, or, infrequently, spur cell anemia [46]. Hemosiderin may be evident in either Kupffer cells, periportal hepatocytes, or both on routine and iron (Prussian blue) stains. Hepatocellular hemosiderosis is typically mild, but once cirrhosis has developed the considerable secondary iron overload may closely mimic that seen in hereditary hemochromatosis. In such cases there is extensive hemosiderin in hepatocytes distributed throughout the nodules, with or without Kupffer cell hemosiderin. The absence of significant hemosiderin in portal tracts, fibrous septa, and bile ducts [47] is helpful in recognizing this as secondary iron overload. The marked elevations of hepatic iron concentration and iron index contribute to the potential diagnostic confusion with hereditary hemochromatosis [47,48]. In the alcoholic without cirrhosis, the presence of moderate periportal hemosiderosis should prompt consideration of obtaining a gene test for hemochromatosis.

Pathologic differential diagnosis

Steatosis and steatohepatitis have a number of different causes other than alcohol (Box 2). In the case of steatosis alone, the differential diagnosis de-

---

Box 2. Pathologic differential diagnosis of steatosis and steatohepatitis

Steatosis
- Macrovesicular
  - Alcohol
  - Obesity
  - Diabetes
  - Hyperlipidemia
  - Corticosteroid therapy
  - Protein–calorie malnutrition
- Microvesicular
  - Alcoholic foamy degeneration
  - Drug hepatotoxicity (eg, nucleoside analogs)
  - Acute fatty liver of pregnancy
  - Urea cycle defects
  - Mitochondriopathies

Steatohepatitis
- Alcoholic steatohepatitis (ASH)
- Nonalcoholic steatohepatitis (NASH)
  - Obesity
  - Diabetes
  - Hyperlipidemia
  - Insulin resistance/metabolic syndrome
  - Drug hepatotoxicity (eg, tamoxifen, nifedipine)

---

pends on the nature of the fat (ie, macrovesicular versus microvesicular). Macrovesicular fat is the form most often encountered in liver biopsy material, and its causes represent common conditions such as obesity, diabetes, and corticosteroid therapy. In contrast, microvesicular steatosis is infrequently present, and is indicative of more serious liver injury in which mitochondrial β-oxidation is affected. Examples of this are small droplet steatosis due to nucleoside reverse transcriptase inhibitors used in the therapy of AIDS [49] and, more classically, acute fatty liver of pregnancy [50].

For steatohepatitis the differential diagnosis rests between ASH and NASH. The latter has a number of causes (Box 2) that require clinical documentation. Pathologic distinction between ASH and NASH on purely morphologic grounds is difficult. This issue was addressed in a comparative study by Diehl et al [51], which identified overlapping features between the two conditions, but also suggested which features might be weighted in favor of one or the other etiology. In general, abundant neutrophils and many Mallory bodies are features favoring alcohol, while substantial macrovesicular steatosis and lymphocytic infiltrates support NAFLD. There are, of course, exceptions to these broad distinctions, and clinical correlation is critical in determining the cause of steatohepatitis.

References

[1] Mallory FB. Cirrhosis of the liver. Five different types of lesions from which it may arise. Bull Johns Hopkins Hosp 1911;22:69–74.

[2] French SW, Nash J, Shitabata P, et al. Pathology of alcoholic liver disease. Semin Liver Dis 1993;13:154–69.

[3] Baptista A, Bianchi L, De Groote J, et al. Alcoholic liver disease: morphological manifestations. Lancet 1981;1:707–11.

[4] Denk H, Stumptner C, Zatloukal K. Mallory bodies revisited. J Hepatol 2000;32:689–702.

[5] Ishak KG, Zimmerman HJ, Ray MB. Alcoholic liver disease: pathologic, pathogenetic and clinical aspects. Alcohol Clin Exp Res 1991;15:45–66.

[6] Friedman SL. Liver fibrosis—from bench to bedside. J Hepatol 2003;38:S38–53.

[7] Hoyumpa AM, Greene HL, Dunn GD, et al. Fatty liver: biochemical and clinical considerations. Dig Dis 1975;20:1142–70.

[8] Sabesin SM, Ragland JB, Freeman MR. Lipoprotein disturbances in liver disease. In: Popper H, Schaffner F, editors. Progress in liver diseases, vol. VI. Orlando: Grune and Stratton; 1979. p. 243–62.

[9] Casini A. Alcohol-induced fatty liver and inflammation: where do Kupffer cells act? J Hepatol 2000;32:1026–30.

[10] Tilg H, Diehl AM. Cytokines in alcoholic and nonalcoholic steatohepatitis. N Engl J Med 2000;343:1467–76.

[11] Washington K, Wright K, Shyr Y, et al. Hepatic stellate cell activation in nonalcoholic steatohepatitis and fatty liver. Hum Pathol 2000;31:822–8.

[12] Angulo P. Nonalcoholic fatty liver disease. N Engl J Med 2002;346:1221–31.

[13] Niemelä O, Parkkila S, Ylä-Herttuala S, et al. Covalent protein adducts in the liver as a result of ethanol metabolism and lipid peroxidation. Lab Invest 1994;70:537–46.

[14] Mavrelis PC, Ammon HV, Gleysteen JJ, et al. Hepatic free fatty acids in alcoholic liver disease and morbid obesity. Hepatology 1983;3:226–31.

[15] Maher J. The CYP2E1 knockout delivers another punch: first ASH, now NASH. Hepatology 2001;33:311–2.

[16] Day CP. Apoptosis in alcoholic hepatitis: a novel therapeutic target? J Hepatol 2001;34: 330–3.

[17] Rust C, Gores GJ. Apoptosis and liver disease. Am J Med 2000;108:567–74.

[18] Uchida T, Kao H, Quispe-Sjogren M, et al. Alcoholic foamy degeneration—a pattern of acute alcoholic injury of the liver. Gastroenterology 1983;84:683–92.

[19] Suri S, Mitros FA, Ahluwalia JP. Alcoholic foamy degeneration and markedly elevated GGT. A case report and literature review. Dig Dis Sci 2003;48:1142–6.

[20] Matteoni CA, Younossi ZM, Gramlich T, et al. Nonalcoholic fatty liver disease: a spectrum of clinical and pathological severity. Gastroenterology 1999;116:1413–9.

[21] Christoffersen P, Braendstrup O, Juhl E, et al. Lipogranulomas in human liver biopsies with fatty change. A morphological, biochemical and clinical investigation. Acta Pathol Microbiol Scand [A] 1971;79:150–8.

[22] Bruguera M, Bertran A, Bombi JA, et al. Giant mitochondria in hepatocytes: a diagnostic hint for alcoholic liver disease. Gastroenterology 1977;73:1383–7.

[23] Caldwell SH, Swerdlow RH, Khan EM, et al. Mitochondrial abnormalities in non-alcoholic steatohepatitis. J Hepatol 1999;31:430–4.

[24] Junge J, Horn T, Christoffersen P. Megamitochondria as a diagnostic marker for alcohol induced centrilobular and periportal fibrosis in the liver. Virchows Arch A Pathol Anat Histopathol 1987;410:553–8.

[25] Ludwig J, Viggiano TR, McGill DB, et al. Nonalcoholic steatohepatitis: Mayo Clinic experiences with a hitherto unnamed disease. Mayo Clin Proc 1980;55:434–8.

[26] Van Eyken P, Sciot R, Desmet VJ. A cytokeratin immunohistochemical study of alcoholic liver disease: evidence that hepatocytes can express "bile duct-type" cytokeratins. Histopathology 1988;13:605–17.

[27] Stumptner C, Omary MB, Fickert P, et al. Hepatocyte cytokeratins are hyperphosphorylated at multiple sites in human alcoholic hepatitis and in a Mallory body mouse model. Am J Pathol 2000;156:77–90.

[28] Stumptner C, Fuchsbichler A, Heid H, et al. Mallory body—a disease-associated type of sequestosome. Hepatology 2002;35:1053–62.

[29] Stumptner C, Heid H, Fuchsbichler A, et al. Analysis of intracytoplasmic hyaline bodies in a hepatocellular carcinoma. Demonstration of p62 as major constituent. Am J Pathol 1999;154:1701–10.

[30] Lefkowitch JH, Haythe JH, Regent N. Kupffer cell aggregation and perivenular distribution in steatohepatitis. Mod Pathol 2002;15:699–704.

[31] Kishi M, Maeyama S, Iwaba A, et al. Hepatic veno-occlusive lesions and other histopathological changes of the liver in severe alcoholic hepatitis—a comparative clinicohistopathological study of autopsy cases. Alcohol Clin Exp Res 2000;24:74S–80S.

[32] Russell RM, Boyer JL, Bagheri SA, et al. Hepatic injury from chronic hypervitaminosis A resulting in portal hypertension and ascites. N Engl J Med 1974;291:435–40.

[33] Latry P, Bioulac-Sage P, Echinard E, et al. Perisinusoidal fibrosis and basement membrane-like material in the livers of diabetic patients. Hum Pathol 1987;18:775–80.

[34] Colombat M, Charlotte F, Ratziu V, et al. Portal lymphocytic infiltrate in alcoholic liver disease. Hum Pathol 2002;33:1170–4.

[35] Van Waes L, Lieber CS. Early perivenular sclerosis in alcoholic fatty liver: an index of progressive liver injury. Gastroenterology 1977;73:646–50.

[36] Mathurin P, Duchatelle V, Ramond MJ, et al. Survival and prognostic factors in patients with severe alcoholic hepatitis treated with prednisolone. Gastroenterology 1996;110:1847–53.

[37] Desmet VJ, Gerber M, Hoofnagle JH, et al. Classification of chronic hepatitis: diagnosis, grading and staging. Hepatology 1994;19:1513–20.

[38] Brunt EM. Grading and staging the histopathological lesions of chronic hepatitis: the Knodell histology activity index and beyond. Hepatology 2000;31:241–6.

[39] Ishak K, Baptista A, Bianchi L, et al. Histological grading and staging of chronic hepatitis. J Hepatol 1995;22:696–9.

[40] Scheuer PJ. Assessment of liver biopsies in chronic hepatitis: how is it best done? J Hepatol 2003;38:240–2.

[41] Brunt EM, Janney CG, Di Bisceglie AM, et al. Nonalcoholic steatohepatitis: a proposal for grading and staging the histological lesions. Am J Gastroenterol 1999;94:2467–74.

[42] Rosman AS, Waraich A, Galvin K, et al. Alcoholism is associated with hepatitis C but not hepatitis B in an urban population. Am J Gastroenterol 1996;91:498–505.

[43] Caldwell SH, Jeffers LJ, Ditomaso A, et al. Antibody to hepatitis C is common among patients with alcoholic liver disease with and without risk factors. Am J Gastroenterol 1991;86:1219–23.

[44] Mendenhall CL, Seeff L, Diehl AM, et al. Antibodies to hepatitis B virus and hepatitis C virus in alcoholic hepatitis and cirrhosis: their prevalence and clinical relevance. Hepatology 1991;14:581–9.

[45] Afroudakis A, Kaplowitz N. Liver histopathology in chronic common bile duct stenosis due to chronic alcoholic pancreatitis. Hepatology 1981;1:65–72.

[46] Pascoe A, Kerlin P, Steadman C, et al. Spur cell anaemia and hepatic iron stores in patients with alcoholic liver disease undergoing orthotopic liver transplantation. Gut 1999;45:301–5.

[47] Deugnier Y, Turlin B, Le Quilleuc D, et al. A reappraisal of hepatic siderosis in patients with end-stage cirrhosis: practical implications for the diagnosis of hemochromatosis. Am J Surg Pathol 1997;21:669–75.

[48] Ludwig J, Hashimoto E, Porayko MK, et al. Hemosiderosis in cirrhosis: a study of 447 native livers. Gastroenterology 1997;112:882–8.

[49] Spengler U, Lichterfeld M, Rockstroh JK. Antiretroviral drug toxicity—a challenge for the hepatologist? J Hepatol 2002;36:283–94.
[50] Rolfes DB, Ishak KG. Acute fatty liver of pregnancy: a clinicopathologic study of 35 cases. Hepatology 1985;5:1149–58.
[51] Diehl AM, Goodman Z, Ishak KG. Alcohollike liver disease in nonalcoholics. A clinical and histologic comparison with alcohol-induced liver injury. Gastroenterology 1988;95: 1056–62.

ELSEVIER
SAUNDERS

Clin Liver Dis 9 (2005) 55–66

CLINICS IN
LIVER DISEASE

Immunology of Alcoholic Liver Disease

Carroll B. Leevy, MD*, Hany A. Elbeshbeshy, MD

*University of Medicine and Dentistry of New Jersey–Newark, New Jersey Medical School,
Liver Center, Sammy Davis Jr. National Liver Institute, 150 Bergen Street, P.O. Box 1709,
Newark, NJ 07101-1709, USA*

The spontaneous transformation of alcoholic-induced fatty liver and alcoholic hepatitis into cirrhosis and liver cancer, despite withdrawal of alcoholic beverages and provision of a nutritious diet, reflects the fact that immunologic hyperactivity is responsible for progressive destruction of hepatocytes and development of cirrhosis in patients with alcoholic hepatitis [1]. This explains the frequent progression of alcoholic hepatitis despite cessation of alcohol intake in some patients [2,3]. Serial studies of patients with alcoholic hepatitis revealed that with continued alcoholism, 80% of such patients develop cirrhosis. In this report, it was suggested that immunologic abnormalities contributed to the development of cirrhosis, and concluded that genetic or acquired deficits alter reactivity of the immune system in alcoholics and lead to neutrophil chemotaxis, cytotoxicity, and fibrogenesis. Direct toxic effects of ethanol or its metabolites on liver may induce neoantigens. Recognition of these neoantigens by T and B cells leads to antibody production with polymorphnuclear leucocyte-induced necrosis characteristic of alcoholic hepatitis [4].

Liver cell damage in alcoholic hepatitis is mediated by disturbances of the immune system, inducing a myriad of immunologic manifestations, which range from activation of macrophage with release of chemokines and pro-inflamatory cytokines like tumor necrosis factor-alpha (TNF-α), IL-1beta, interleukin-6 (IL-6), interleukin-8 (IL-8), and transforming growth factor β to lymphocyte function depression. Chronic alcohol exposure increases the influx of endotoxins from the gut into the portal circulation, and formation of malondialdehyde–aldehyde protein adducts, both processes that can then lead to increased expression of cell adhesion molecules and cytokine production

* Corresponding author.
E-mail address: leevycb@umdnj.edu (C.B. Leevy).

1089-3261/05/$ – see front matter © 2005 Elsevier Inc. All rights reserved.
doi:10.1016/j.cld.2004.11.002

by Kupffer cells and sinusoidal endothelial cells. Liver-associated T lympho-cytes mediate injury, both by immune-mediated and nonimmune-mediated he-patic injury.

Several obligatory features define the lesion of alcoholic hepatitis: liver cell necrosis, perivenular distribution, pericellular fibrosis, and infiltration by neutrophils and hyaline bodies. The latter has had attention focused on by sev-eral groups as the factor responsible for the immune reactions observed in alcoholic hepatitis [4].

Neutrophil accumulation is relatively unique to alcoholic injury (in most forms of hepatitis, mononuclear cells predominate), and may contribute to hepa-tocellular injury. Neutrophil infiltration/activity may occur through release of neutrophil chemoattractants by hepatocytes metabolizing ethanol. Tissue injury could ensue from neutrophils and hepatocytes releasing reactive oxygen inter-mediates, proteases, and cytokines.

In alcoholic liver disease (ALD) the number of lymphocytes in the liver increases and the type and distribution of these infiltrating cells will determine the nature of the inflammation. For instance, a predominance of parenchymal inflammation is a feature of alcoholic hepatitis, whereas a predominantly portal infiltrate is a feature of cirrhosis.

Lymphocytes play a critical role in regulating the immune/inflammatory response to alcohol. Although the inflammatory cell infiltrate is predominantly neutrophils, both CD4-positive and CD8-positive lymphocytes are also detected.

Kupffer cells

Liver macrophages

Kupffer cells (Fig. 1), reticuloendothelial cells in the walls of the sinusoids of the liver, were described by Kupffer, a German anatomist, in 1876. His observations led to a better understanding of the so-called reticuloendothelial (macrophage) system. The Kupffer cells belong to the group of mixed macrophages. They act to clear the blood of foreign particles, aging and damaged red blood cells, and other cellular debris. They are also said to play a role in fat metabolism, conservation of iron, and in the formation of bile pigment.

The role of Kupffer cells in initiating the inflammatory process of alcoholic hepatitis

Chronic alcohol intake increases gut permeability, which results in increased levels of Lipopolysaccharide (LPS) in the peripheral circulation. LPS binds with LPS-binding protein (LBP) to make a LPS–LBP complex that binds to CD14 receptors on Kupffer cells. This LPS–CD14 complex further interacts with Toll-like receptor 4, which transduces signals to the cytoplasm that results in an activation of nuclear factor-kappa B (NFκB).

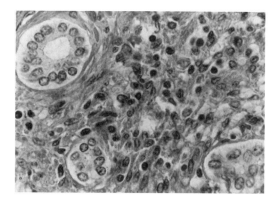

Fig. 1. Kupffer cells.

LPS-stimulated Kupffer cells can also activate NFκB by means of oxidant stress. Activated NFκB binds to nuclear elements, and the outcome is upregulation of proinflamatory cytokines (eg, TNF-α, IL-6, IL-8) and cyclooxygenase-2, which initiate a cascade of inflammatory events that may lead to hepatitis [5,6].

Neutrophils

One of the most characteristic pathologic hallmarks of alcoholic hepatitis is infiltration of neutrophils, which are generally absent from other forms of inflammatory liver disease, generally in association with an increase in the peripheral neutrophil count.

IL-8 is a member of the chemokine family, and a known neutrophil chemo-attractant. Elevated plasma IL-8 levels have been documented in patients with alcoholic hepatitis. The plasma IL-8 levels correlated with the severity of hepatic injury, and IL-8 has been identified immunohistochemically in the liver in alcoholic patients.

Whether IL-8 is produced locally in the liver and is required for injury to occur is unproven [7,8].

Potential mechanisms by which neutrophils damage hepatocytes in alcoholic hepatitis involve two steps: attachment of neutrophils to hepatocytes, and neutrophil-induced cytotoxicity [9,10].

Lymphocytes

Studies were undertaken to evaluate the cytotoxicity of peripheral lymphocytes obtained from patients with ALD. Lymphocyte cytotoxicity to the Chang liver cells was investigated, and that to autologous liver cells obtained by percutaneous liver biopsy. Lymphocytes from patients with alcoholic liver

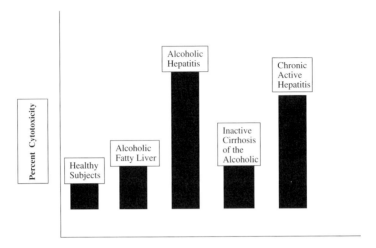

Fig. 2. Cytotoxic effects on Chang liver cells of lymphocytes from healthy subjects and from patients with ALD or chronic active hepatitis.

hepatitis were found to be highly cytotoxic to Chang liver cells and autologous liver cells when compared with those of healthy subjects (Fig. 2).

In one study, preincubation of sensitized lymphocytes with acetaldehyde increased cytotoxicity for autologous liver beyond that obtained by the combined effects of lymphocytes alone and acetaldehyde alone, interpreted as evidence that ethanol toxicity and hyperactivity of lymphocytes independently and collectively contribute to development of cirrhosis in patients with alcoholic hepatitis who continue to imbibe alcohol [2] (Fig. 3).

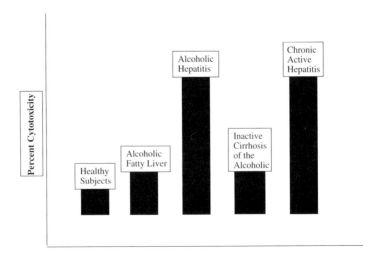

Fig. 3. Cytotoxic effects of lymphocytes on autologous liver cells from healthy subjects and from patients with ALD or chronic active hepatitis.

Cytotoxicity

Lymphocytes are responsible for cytotoxic reactions encountered in liver disease, where both T and B lymphocytes may cause cell lysis. Activation of cytotoxic lymphocytes requires the participation of macrophages, which function as nonspecific accessory cells.

Fibrogenesis

Of equal importance to cytotoxicity in the development of chronic liver disease is collagen deposition and scar formation. In one study where supernatants of hyperactive lymphocytes were added to either cultured fibroblasts or autologous liver cells, this caused a significant increase in collagen secretion by microtubules [11] (Fig. 3).

The possible mechanisms by which lymphocytes are recruited to the liver during alcoholic hepatitis

Lymphocyte's role in causing injury to hepatocytes in alcoholic hepatitis has been shown by examination of liver biopsy samples obtained from patients with ALD, which revealed the presence of increased numbers of CD4 and CD8 T cells. The ratio of CD8/CD4 T cells is higher in liver than in peripheral blood. These lymphocytes, when stimulated by endotoxins, are capable of causing apoptosis and necrosis of hepatocytes by increasing the production of inflammatory cytokines (eg, TNF-α) and free radicals such as nitric oxide.

There is another possible mechanism by which lymphocytes, sequestered in a liver affected with alcoholic hepatitis, cause damage to hepatocytes. The lymphocyte plasma membrane makes focal point contacts with the hepatocyte plasma membrane forming the immunologic synapse, resulting in an enhanced expression of class II major histocompatability complex molecules by hepatocytes. This is followed by the internalization of the immunologic synapse complex components through lymphocyte plasma membrane receptor-mediated endocytosis. The lysosomal enzymes digest these internalized complexes. This process is repeated until the target cell is completely digested by the lymphocytes. This leads to progressive liver cell loss and subsequent replacement by collagen that results in fibrosis [9,12].

Immune complexes

Immune complexes are found in acute and chronic viral hepatitis, primary biliary, cirrhosis, and alcoholic hepatitis. The properties of these complexes vary greatly, depending upon antigen and antibody levels and the use of complements. They may be detected in both serum and tissue of patients with

Table 1
Immune complexes in liver from patients with alcoholic hepatitis

Diagnosis	Immunoglobulins in mg/100 Gm liver			I.A. Titre of elute
	IgG	IgA	IgM	
Advanced alcoholic Hepatitis (3)	0.18–0.66	0–0.5	0	32–256
Active alcoholic Cirrhosis (3)	0.15–2.3	0–0.3	0	256–512
Inactive alcoholic Cirrhosis (3)	0.15–0.72	0	0	0
Controls (2)	0	0–0.6	0	0

alcoholic hepatitis. Immunoglobulin eluted from the liver of patients dying of severe alcoholic hepatitis were active against hyaline bodies (Table 1).

The demonstration of immune complexes explains the frequent systemic manifestations seen in liver disease, including skin rashes, cutaneous hemorrhages, arthralgia, proteinuria, renal failure, thrombocytopenia, and hypocomplementemia.

The deposition of immune complexes in acute and chronic active hepatitis leads to complement-mediated antibody cytotoxicity. Immune complexes are, therefore, of key importance to the development of hepatic necrosis [11].

Hyaline bodies

A hyaline body is a cytoplasmic substance without a membrane enclosure, which appears as pinkish structureless material in hematoxylin-eosin stained sections. It primarily occurs in hepatocytes located in the centrilobular area, but may also be seen in ductular or sinusoidal cells. Histochemically, it contains protein, carbohydrate, lipid, and ribonucleic acid. It is synthesized by ribosomes, and is an actin-like, relatively insoluble protein (Fig. 4).

Mallory postulated that hyaline seen in postmortem specimens of alcoholic hepatitis is responsible for liver necrosis, polymorphnuclear inflammation, and fibrosis [11].

It has been found that hyaline bodies are released into the circulation where it evokes both humoral and cell-mediated immunity [13]. Hyaline bodies consist of five distinct fractions, each of which exhibits antigenic activity in experimental animals [14]. Once it is formed, it is released into circulation, where it stimulates B cells to produce antibodies. Serum alcoholic hyaline antibody (AHAb) and antigen (AHAg) have been detected in patients with alcoholic hepatitis using the immune hemagglutinin test. Lymphokines released from lymphocytes sensitized to hyaline bodies include blastogenic, cytotoxic, migration inhibition, chemotactic, and fibrogenic factors. Subsequent events are determined by the amount of circulating hyaline and host responsiveness. It has been found that ethanol and hyaline bodies are synergistic in inducing fibrogenesis. Hyaline body-sensitized lymphocytes preincubated with acetal-

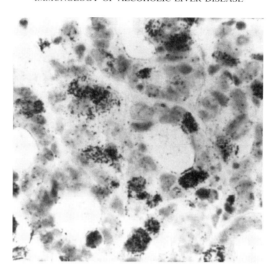

Fig. 4. Inflammation and hyaline bodies are present in alcoholic hepatitis. Hyaline bodies are cytoplasmic, eosinophilic, rope-like inclusions within the cytoplasm of hepatocytes.

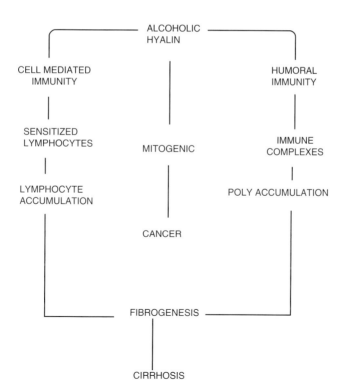

Fig. 5. Potential immunopathologic effects of hyaline bodies (alcoholic hyalin).

dehyde exhibit a significantly greater cytotoxicity to autologous liver cells. This observation explains progressive liver cell necrosis found in patients with alcoholic hepatitis who continue to consume alcohol. Patients with early-phase alcoholic hepatitis often have circulating AHAg. Patients with severe alcoholic hepatitis usually exhibit positive AHAb or circulating immune complexes [15] (Fig. 5).

Chemokines

Chemokines are responsible for the attraction of leukocytes, adhesion molecules that promote the attachment of leukocytes to the endothelial cells and hepatocytes.

Chemokines belong to a large family of small chemotactic cytokines [16,17]. Chemokines are widely expressed and involved in many biologic processes. They exert their biologic effects by binding to complementary G-protein–coupled receptors expressed on the target cells. Chemokines secreted at a particular site can be concentrated on vessels in that tissue by sequestration on endothelial glycosaminoglycans, which provides a mechanism for the presentation of lo-cally secreted chemokines from several sources to the circulating leukocyte. Activation of chemokine receptors on adherent leukocytes leads to signaling and activation of integrins and cytoskeletal reorganization [18].

Tumor necrosis factor-alpha

It is clear that cytokines cause metabolic disturbances that are similar to known complications of ALD. TNF-α appears to be a proximal mediator of multiple types of experimental liver injury, and TNF-α activity is elevated in ALD, as are the levels of certain other cytokines. Alternatively, low physiologic amounts of cytokines appear to be important for liver regeneration, and perhaps are beneficial to the organ as a whole [19].

Blood levels of TNF-α and IgA are increased in patients with ALD. IgA stimulates TNF-α secretion by monocytes from patients with ALD.

There is a significant positive correlations between expression of IgA and TNF-α. These findings in acute alcoholic hepatitis could be the result of activation of Kupffer cells by IgA in portal venous blood to produce TNF-α, which in turn, induces apoptosis in adjacent hepatocytes [20].

There are various molecular pathways that mediate the cytotoxic effects of TNF-α on the hepatic parenchymal cells. The effects of TNF-α on liver cells are mediated through two types of plasma membrane receptors: p55 (type 1 tumor necrosis factor receptor [TNFR1]) and p75 (type 2 tumor necrosis fac-tor receptor [TNFR2]), of which TNFR1 predominates in the liver cells. Binding of TNF-α with TNFR1 activates signaling pathways, leading to apoptosis, necrosis, or cytoprotective effects. One apoptotic pathway involves proteins such as TNF-α receptor-associated death domain protein and Fas-activated death domain protein, which activate caspase 8, whereas another pathway involves receptor-interacting protein and TNF-α receptor-associated factor. The cytoprotective pathway probably also involves receptor-interacting protein and TNF-α receptor-associated factor, leading to NFκB activation, which increases the transcription of the genes of inhibitors of apoptosis.

In addition to TNF-α, a role has emerged for cyclooxygenase 2. This enzyme, which produces prostaglandins, is elevated in experimental alcoholic liver injury, raising the possibility that inhibitors may have a therapeutic benefit [21,22].

Interleukin-6

IL-6 is a fibrogenic cytokine with multiple biologic activities. Cells known to express IL-6 include CD8 T cells, fibroblasts, endothelial cells, neutrophils, monocytes, and eosinophils. IL-6 production is generally correlated with cell activation. Circulating IL-6 can be found in the blood of normal individuals. It causes lymphocyte activation and antibody release, and hepatocyte release of acute phase reactants. IL-6 has the further effect of suppressing hepatocyte albumin production, associated prospectively with increased mortality [23].

Interleukin-8

IL-8 is a CXC class chemokine, produced by many cell types, including monocytes, fibroblasts, hepatocytes, Kupffer cells, neutrophils, and endothelial cells in response to infection. It promotes migration of neutrophils into surrounding tissue; it is also expressed on endothelial cells in response to inflammation, and binds to IL-8 receptors, which is expressed on neutrophils in response to inflammation.

Patients with alcoholic hepatitis often have hepatic polymorphonuclear leukocyte infiltration and neutrophilia. IL-8 is a cytokine that stimulates neutrophil chemotaxis and release of lysosomal enzymes. Increased IL-8 concentrations in patients with alcoholic hepatitis suggest a role for IL-8 in the neutrophilia and hepatic polymorphonuclear leukocyte infiltration of alcoholic hepatitis [8].

A study that was performed to evaluate the role of IL-8 in the pathogenesis of alcoholic hepatitis, using enzyme-linked immunosorbent assay, measured serum IL-8 levels in patients with alcoholic hepatitis. The mean serum IL-8 level was increased significantly in patients with alcoholic hepatitis compared with normal controls. It was of interest to note that serum IL-8 levels were increased transiently after abstinence from alcohol in patients with alcoholic hepatitis. These findings suggest that there may be a correlation between IL-8 and alcoholic hepatitis [24].

A different study measured IL-8 in patients with a spectrum of ALD and in normal and diseased control subjects. Levels of circulating IL-8 were undetectable in normal subjects but highly elevated in patients with alcoholic hepatitis, particularly in those who died [7].

Antigenic adduct formation

Acetaldehyde and hydroxyethyl radicals are both derived from the oxidation of ethanol, binding valently to proteins, where they form adducts that are antigenic. Acetaldehyde, which is a highly reactive molecule that can bind avidly to the epsilon amino group of internal lysine residues and the alpha amino N-terminal amino acids of proteins, creating acetaldehyde–protein adducts through a Schiff base mechanism.

Two potentially important consequences of adduct formation

1. Adducts could form with intracellular proteins that are critical to cellular function, leading to dysfunction.
2. Acetaldehyde protein adducts may act as neoantigens, provoking both cell-mediated and humoral immune responses to attack cells bearing these compounds.

Several studies have identified antibodies in the serum of alcoholics who are reactive to acetaldehyde adducts; however, this observation does not easily explain how the antibodies might attack an intracellular protein. In addition, acetaldehyde–protein adducts have also been detected in patients with non-ALD.

Hydroxyethyl radical adducts also may play an important role in the pathogenesis of alcohol-induced liver injury [25].

In one report, animals given ethanol in vivo generated hydroxyethyl adducts on the external surface of hepatocytes that were recognized by anti-hydroxyethyl radical adduct antibodies that were present in the sera of cirrhotic patients. In the presence of monocytes, this antigen–antibody complex was able to trigger a cell-mediated cytotoxic reaction that killed the hepatocytes [26,27].

Summary

Alcohol-induced liver injury is a reflection of the immunologic response of the liver to this stimulus. Reported studies of immunologic abnormalities in ALD patients suggest that immunologic response plays a key role in the pathogenesis of chronic liver disease in alcoholics, and have contributed to the understanding of how some patients with ALD progress into alcoholic liver cirrhosis. The immunologic response of the liver is reflected in alcoholic fatty liver, hyaline necrosis, and cirrhosis, promoted by the role of neutrophils in damaging liver cells through cytotoxicity, and lymphocytes through cytotoxicity, inducing fibrogenesis of the liver and formation of immune complexes responsible for immune complex-mediated cytotoxicity, in addition to the role of different chemokines in attracting leucocytes, inducing fibrogenesis and liver cell apoptosis, with the established mechanism by which Mallory bodies evoke both cellular and humoral immunity contributing to the process of alcoholic liver cirrhosis, which plays a key role in transformation of alcoholic hepatitis to cirrhosis. At present, research is underway to find modalities to correct the induced immunologic changes, so at this time, it is necessary to avoid alcoholism, with the use of social and educational programs to stop alcoholism.

References

[1] Zetterman RK, Leevy CM. Immunologic reactivity and alcoholic live disease. Bull NY Acad Med 1975;51(4):533–44.

[2] Shinichi K, Leevy CM. Lymphocyte cytotoxicity alcoholic hepatitis. Gastroenterology 1977;72:594–7.

[3] Leevy CM. Fatty liver: a study of 270 patients with biopsy proven fatty liver and review of the literature. Medicine (Baltimore) 1962;41:249–76.

[4] Kanagasundaram N, Leevy CM. Immunologic aspects of liver disease. Med Clin North Am 1979;63(3):631–42.

[5] Nanji AA. Role of Kupffer cells in alcoholic hepatitis. Alcohol 2002;27(1):13–5.

[6] Nanji AA, Su GL, Laposata M, et al. Pathogenesis of alcoholic liver disease, recent advances. Alcohol Clin Exp Res 2002;26(5):731–6.

[7] Sheron N, Bird G, Koskinas J, et al. Circulating and tissue levels of the neutrophil chemotaxin interleukin-8 are elevated in severe acute alcoholic hepatitis, and tissue levels correlate with neutrophil infiltration. Hepatology 1993;18(1):41–6.

[8] Hill DB, Marsano LS, McClain CJ. Increased plasma interleukin-8 concentrations in alcoholic hepatitis. Hepatology 1993;18(3):576–80.

[9] Purohit V, Russo D. Cellular and molecular mechanisms of alcoholic hepatitis: introduction and summary of the symposium. Alcohol 2002;27(1):3–6.

[10] Jaeschke H. Neutrophil mediated tissue injury in alcoholic hepatitis. Alcohol 2002;27(1):23–7.

[11] Kanagasundaram N, Leevy CM. Immunologic aspects of liver disease. Med Clin North Am 1979;63(3):631–42.

[12] Batey RG, Cao Q, Gould B. Lymphocyte-mediated liver injury in alcohol-related hepatitis. Alcohol 2002;27(1):37–41.

[13] Leevy CM, Chen T, Luisada-Opper A, et al. Liver disease of the alcoholic: role of immunologic abnormalities in pathogenesis, recognition, and treatment. Prog Liver Dis 1976;5:516–30.

[14] Leevy CM, Kanagasundaram N, Leevy CB, et al. Isolation and purification of alcoholic hyaline. In: Preisig R, editor. Proceedings third international Gstaad symposium on the liver. Quantitative aspects of structure and function. Basel (Switzerland): Karger; 1978.

[15] Matsumoto K, Saha A, Leevy CM. Immunochemical studies on alcoholic hyalin. Gastroenterol Jpn 1979;14(6):573–83.

[16] Moser B, Loetscher P. Lymphocyte traffic control by chemokines. Nat Immunol 2001;2(2): 123–8.

[17] Murdoch C, Finn A. Chemokine receptors and their role in inflammation and infectious diseases. Blood 2000;95(10):3032–43.

[18] Haydon G, Lalor PF, Hubscher SG, et al. Lymphocyte recruitment to the liver in alcoholic liver disease. Alcohol 2002;27(1):29–36.

[19] McClain C, Hill D, Schmidt J, et al. Cytokines and alcoholic liver disease. Semin Liver Dis 1993;13(2):170–82.

[20] Deviere J, Vaerman JP, Content J, et al. IgA triggers tumor necrosis factor alpha secretion by monocytes: a study in normal subjects and patients with alcoholic cirrhosis. Hepatology 1991; 13(4):670–5.

[21] Nanji AA, Zakim D, Rahemtulla A, et al. Dietary saturated fatty acids down-regulate cyclooxygenase-2 and tumor necrosis factor alfa and reverse fibrosis in alcohol-induced liver disease in the rat. Hepatology 1997;26(6):1538–45.

[22] Rodriguez DA, Moncada C, Nunez MT, et al. Ethanol increases tumor necrosis factor-alpha receptor-1 (TNF-R1) levels in hepatic, intestinal, and cardiac cells. Alcohol 2004;33(1): 9–15.

[23] Kowalski-Saunders PW, Winwood PJ, Arthur MJ, et al. Reversible inhibition of albumin production by rat hepatocytes maintained on a laminin-rich gel (Engelbreth–Holm–Swarm) in response to secretory products of Kupffer cells and cytokines. Hepatology 1992;16(3): 733–41.

[24] Masumoto T, Onji M, Horiike N, et al. Assay of serum interleukin 8 levels in patients with alcoholic hepatitis. Alcohol Alcohol Suppl 1993;1A:99–102.

[25] Clot P, Parola M, Bellomo G, et al. Plasma membrane hydroxyethyl radical adducts cause antibody-dependent cytotoxicity in rat hepatocytes exposed to alcohol. Gastroenterology 1997;113(1):265–76.

[26] Tuma DJ, Sorrell MF. The role of acetaldehyde adducts in liver injury. Prog Clin Biol Res 1985;183:3–17.

[27] Niemela O, Parkkila S, Yla-Herttuala S, et al. Covalent protein adducts in the liver as a result of ethanol metabolism and lipid peroxidation. Lab Invest 1994;70(4):537–46.

ELSEVIER
SAUNDERS

CLINICS IN
LIVER DISEASE

Clin Liver Dis 9 (2005) 67–81

Nutritional Aspects of Alcoholic Liver Disease

Carroll M. Leevy, MD*, Şerban A. Moroianu, MD

*University of Medicine & Dentistry of New Jersey, 150 Bergen Street, Room H-245,
Newark, NJ 07101-1709, USA*

Alcoholic liver disease is usually associated with clinical and laboratory evidence of nutritional deficiency. These are clinical and laboratory evidence of vitamin, mineral, and protein deficiencies associated with fatty liver, alcoholic hepatitis, and cirrhosis attributable to decreased intake, malabsorption, maluse, and increased loss of essential nutrients. These patients have progressive changes in nutrient status as the hepatic disease worsens; only cessation of alcohol intake will allow restoration of normal nutritional status. Unfortunately, the depleted patient exhibits mental abnormalities, which may prevent adherence to an alcohol-free dietary intake.

Effects of ethanol on vitamin transport, use, and metabolism

Alcoholism leads to vitamin deficiency because of defects in absorption reflected by low serum vitamin levels (Fig. 1), decreased storage of ingested vitamins, and a decreased ability to convert them into metabolically active forms (Fig. 2).

Retinol (vitamin A)

Mean plasma retinol levels tend to be significantly decreased in alcoholic patients with liver cirrhosis compared with controls [1]. Although the primary

* Corresponding author.
E-mail address: leevycm@umdnj.edu (C.M. Leevy).

1089-3261/05/$ – see front matter © 2005 Elsevier Inc. All rights reserved.
doi:10.1016/j.cld.2004.11.003
liver.theclinics.com

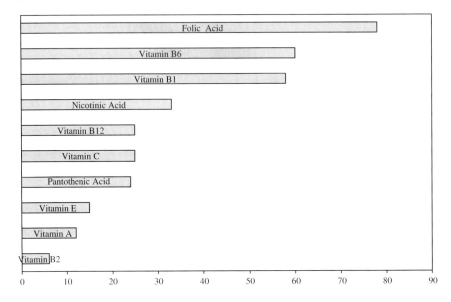

Fig. 1. Circulating vitamin levels in alcoholics with fatty liver and cirrhosis. (*Data from* Leevy CM. Alcoholic liver disease. Clinician-2. Yale Medical School's Gerald Klaskin.)

mechanism appears to be the inadequate intake, there are studies showing that failing plasma levels indicate exhaustion of its hepatic storage [2], and it is therefore suggested that this should be given along with other vitamins during detoxification to prevent hypovitaminosis A [3].

Retinol (vitamin A) must be metabolized to retinoic acid to carry out its role in reproduction, growth, and epithelial development. The enzymes involved in this process are the same enzymes that are metabolizing the ethanol to acetate. Retinol is oxidized to retinal by members of the alcohol dehydrogenase (ADH) family, followed by oxidation of retinal to the active ligand, retinoic, by aldehyde dehydrogenases (ALDHs). Retinoic acid controls the retinoic acid receptor signaling pathways, where receptors function by directly interacting with DNA regulatory sequences leading to modulation of gene transcription [4].

The potential dual role of ALDH and ADH in both ethanol and retinol metabolism provides a common pathway through which disruption in metabolism of one substrate may affect the metabolism of the other. Specifically, inhibition of retinoic acid synthesis, and hence disruption, of retinoid signaling resulting in interference in gene regulation, are a likely mechanism of ethanol-related injury [5].

Vitamin A deficiencies appear to be responsible for alcohol-related disorders such as night blindness and impaired immune function [6]. Supplementation in alcoholic patients may not only correct night blindness and sexual impotence, but may also alleviate liver dysfunction [7].

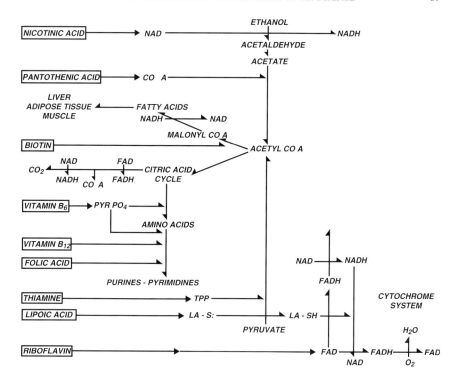

Fig. 2. The biochemical interference of alcohol in metabolism of various vitamins. (*Adapted from* Leevy CM, Barber H, et al. B-complex vitamins in liver disease of the alcoholic. Am J Clin Nutr 1965, with permission.)

It appears that ethanol [8,9], drugs that induce cytochrome P450 in the liver [10], and other xenobiotics that are known to interact with liver microsomes, including carcinogens, causes depletion of hepatic vitamin A, which is exacerbated when these factors are combined [11].

Hepatic vitamin A depletion plays an important role in hepatic fibrosis. A decrease of vitamin A storage in hepatic stellate cells may be associated with the activation of these cells into myofibroblast-like cells, which than can synthesize collagen. Vitamin A deficiency was associated with a number of abnormalities, such as an increasing the risk of esophageal cancer [12].

Equally important are the manifestations related to an excess of vitamin A in alcoholics who continue the drinking habit. Hypervitaminosis A in the presence of ethanol leads to specific lesions such as giant mitochondria (Fig. 3) containing "paracrystaline" filamentous inclusions [13].

It has been shown that although up to five times the daily vitamin A has no detectable adverse effects when given alone, when combined with alcohol, there is a significant leakage of the mitochondrial enzyme glutamic dehydrogenase into the blood stream. This increases the potential hepatic fibrosis. High inci-

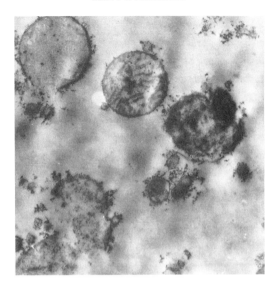

Fig. 3. Enlarged mitochondria as a result of hypervitaminosis A in the presence of ethanol.

dence of squamous cell carcinoma of the lung was found in a Norwegian population that drank large amounts of alcohol and had alcoholic cirrhosis with low dietary intake of vitamin A [56].

Vitamin B complex

Clinical stigmata of B-complex vitamin deficiency, abnormal vitamin levels in biologic fluids, and decreased conversion of free vitamins into coenzymes are often present in malnourished alcoholics with liver disease. Such alterations appear to be of major importance in perpetuating liver injury and interfering with its repair. This thesis has led to wide clinical use of B-complex vitamins for patients with liver disease.

Vitamin B_1 (thiamine)

Thiamine deficiency appears to be the most common and possibly the most important cause of tissue damage in alcoholic patients. Thiamine deficiency is primarily due to interference of ethanol with the gastrointestinal absorption of thiamine and synthesis of coenzyme and thiamine-dependent halo enzymes [15].

Thiamine metabolism is profoundly altered by: (a) decreased formation of thiamine pyrophosphate due to diminished availability of ATP; (b) reduced transketolase or pyruvate decarboxylase activity; (c) absence of substrate for appropriate enzyme activity.

Thiamine deficiency is responsible for Wernicke encephalopathy (which usually responds to administration of thiamine when folate, vitamin B_{12} and protein levels are normal) [16]. Alcoholic polyneuropathy appears to be caused by a defect in thiamine use. Alcoholics with liver disease have lower levels of circulating vitamin B1 than alcoholics with normal liver histology [17].

Vitamin B_2 (riboflavin)

The low intake of vitamin B in alcoholic patients is associated with a relative riboflavin deficiency. Experiments show that ethanol decreases riboflavin storage in experimental animals [18].

Vitamin B_3 (niacin)

Alcoholics often manifest niacin deficiency, which may cause pellagra. In addition, vitamin B_3 deficiency often exists in the absence of the skin lesions, which are characteristic in pellagra. A study published by Ishii and Nishihara [19,20] revealed that in 20 alcoholic patients evidence of pellagra was found at autopsy. These patients had entered the hospital confused, disoriented, and agitated. The typical pellagra skin lesions were absent. Treatment with vitamins B_1, B_6, B_{12}, and C was unsuccessful. Later, diarrhea occurred. They failed to respond to treatment, and died from bronchopneumonia. Subsequently, four other patients presented in similar fashion, niacin was added to the therapeutic regimen, and each recovered.

Vitamin B_6 (pyridoxine)

Neurologic, hematologic, and dermatologic disorders in alcoholic patient can be caused in part by pyridoxine deficiency. A depletion of vitamin B_6, reflected by low plasma levels of pyridoxal 5'-phosphate was reported in over 50% of alcoholics without hematologic findings or abnormal liver function tests. Reduced plasma levels of pyridoxal 5' phosphate are explained, on one hand, by an inadequate intake, as well as by increased destruction in erythrocytes in the presence of acetaldehyde (resulting from ethanol oxidation), and reduced formation on the other [21]. Several studies [22,23] reveal that long-term ethanol abuse lowers hepatic reserves of pyridoxal phosphate.

Vitamin B_{12} (ciancobalamine)

Alcoholics usually exhibit normal levels of circulating levels of cobalamine, this is due in part, to the large body stores of vitamin B_{12} [24]. When these patients, exhibit pancreatic insufficiency associated with liver disease, resulting inadequate absorption of ciancobalamine often causes vitamin B_{12} deficiency [24]. There is also evidence that patients with significant liver damage might have low hepatic resources of cobalamine [25]. Noteworthy is the fact serum levels of cobalamine and its analogs may be normal in serum despite its liver depletion in patients with alcoholism [26].

Folic acid

Alcoholics folate induced typically have low serum and tissue folic acid. Alcohol accelerates the occurrence of megaloblastic anemia. When ingested in large amounts, alcohol causes a decrease in serum folate, which is due in part to its urinary excretion [27], when ethanol is administered chronically, low folate levels are registered due to the inability of the liver to retain folate (Fig. 4) [28].

Vitamin C

Vitamin C deficiency tends to be more frequent in alcoholics than in non-alcoholics this is reflected in decreased serum ascorbic level, in peripheral leukocyte ascorbic acid, or in decreased urinary ascorbic acid after an oral challenge [8,29]. When taken before or during alcohol ingestion, supplementation with ascorbic acid may prevent fatty infiltration of the liver [30].

Vitamin D

Alcoholics may present abnormalities of calcium and phosphorus homeostasis. They may therefore exhibit a decrease in bone density, bone mass, and increased susceptibility to fractures, and evidence of osteonecrosis. These abnormalities result from lack of substrate caused by poor dietary intake, malabsorption due to cholestasis and associated pancreatic insufficiency, and inadequate sunlight exposure.

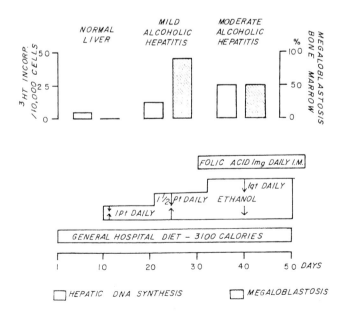

Fig. 4. Influence of ethanol and folate therapy or liver necrosis and regeneration with alcoholism.

Vitamin E

Vitamin E (Alpha tocopherol) diminishes the enhanced peroxidation of lipids that occur during heavy ethanol intake. Vitamin E levels are depressed in patients with alcoholic liver cirrhosis.

Plasma vitamin E levels are significantly lower in those patients who used more than 200 g of ethanol daily (compare with those who used lesser amounts), and in those who presents significant liver damage [31,32]. Plasmatic vitamin E concentrations and vitamin E/total lipid ratio are significantly lower in patients with pancreatitis and a vitamin E/total lipid ratio <1 is routinely associated with steatorrhea [3].

Vitamin K

A deficiency of vitamin K may occur in alcoholism when there is a disruption of fat absorption due to pancreatic insufficiency, biliary obstruction, or structural abnormalities of intestinal mucosa due to folic acid deficiency [24].

Effects of ethanol on absorption and use of minerals

Calcium

Hypocalcaemia, which is frequently seen in alcoholics, is primarily due to hypoalbuminemia, but could also result from vitamin D deficiency, deficient intake, excessive renal loss, malabsorption, as well as from hypomagnesaemia [33]. Low calcium levels are seen in those alcoholics who presents with acute pancreatitis.

Copper

High alcohol intake is associated with higher serum copper levels [34].

Iron

Iron serum levels are elevated in active alcohol drinkers, and tend to normalize with abstinence. Occasional iron deficiency is seen in alcoholism due to gastro-intestinal blood loss, inflammation of gastric mucosa (acute gastritis), or bleeding varices [35].

Magnesium

Hypomagnesaemia, frequently seen in hospitalized patients with alcoholism, is primarily due to deficient intake, but malabsorption, excessive renal loss, and reduced cellular uptake may contribute [33]. This results in intracellular magnesium depletion, which can lead to cardiomyopathy.

Phosphorus

Hyphosphatemia may results from similar causes as mentioned above (for hypomagnesaemia), and when severe, may causes neurologic features similar to those of delirium tremens and visual hallucinations [36–38,64].

Potassium

Potassium plasma levels may be depressed in delirium tremens.

Selenium

Selenium is essential for the activity of glutathione peroxidase, which protects against alcohol-induced liver damage, and its supplementation may benefit patients with alcoholic cirrhosis [20].

Zinc

Chronic ethanol consumption is occasionally associated with zinc deficiency. This is seen in subjects with alcoholic cirrhosis and night blindness who are refractory to vitamin A, given without zinc.

Lithium

Lithium appears to reduce depression in alcoholics and may decrease craving for ethanol [20].

Effects of ethanol on absorption and use of amino acids

Alcohol given in a single customary drink may cause impaired hepatic amino acid uptake, decreased leucine oxidation, and reduced synthesis of lipoproteins, albumin, and fibrinogen [24,39]. When used chronically, ethanol causes impaired secretion of protein due to structural alterations in microtubules and sequestration of proteins in enlarged hepatic cells [24,40].

Arginine

In experimental in vitro studies, arginine was found to interact with acetaldehyde, the metabolite of ethanol, involved in alcohol toxicity [41].

L-glutamine

L-glutamine is one of the factors involved in reducing craving for alcohol. In a double-blind crossover study two groups of 10 patients, each with a long history of excessive consumption of ethanol, took five capsules with meals of either 0.2 g L-glutamine or lactose (as placebo). After 6 weeks, 9 out of 10 patients on L-glutamine exhibited a reduction in desire for drinking alcohol. In contrast, in the placebo group there was no alteration [42].

Glycine and serine

Glycine and serine appear to be involved in reducing acute ethanol intoxication due to a decrease in the rate of absorption of ethanol [43].

Methionine

Methionine deficiency has been described, especially in patients with long-term alcohol consumption who exhibit enhanced use of this amino acid. Inclusion of methionine in the supplementation therapy in those with alcoholic liver disease, has been beneficial. Excess methionine, however, has been shown to produce side effects such as decrease in hepatic adenosine triphosphate. A delay in the clearance of plasma methionine is noted after its systemic administration to patients with liver damage [44].

A significant amount of methionine is metabolized by the liver, patients with hepatic disease exhibit impaired metabolism of this amino acid. For most of its functions, methionine must be activated to S-adenosyl methionine (SAM) [21]. In patients with hepatic cirrhosis, there is a significant decrease in methionine adenosyl amino transferase (also known as S-adenosyl methionine synthetase) [21,40].

A major contribution in inactivation of this enzyme has been relative hypoxia, which is responsible for nitric oxide inactivation and transcriptional arrest [45]. SAM depletion may induce cellular membrane injury, due to the fact that SAM is the principal methylating agent in transmethylation reactions, which are responsible for membranar fluidity and transmembranar transport and transmission of signals [21].

In addition, due to the fact that SAM plays an important role in synthesis of cystheine for glutathione and other polyamines, the deficiency in methionine activation and production of SAM is a major cause of cysteine and glutathione deficiency in alcoholic patients [24].

Clinical trials reveal that SAM is beneficial in treating intrahepatic cholestasis. Moreover, there appears to be a significant improvement in survival and delayed need for liver transplantation in patients with alcoholic cirrhosis treated with SAM [46].

Taurine

Taurine has proven to be a potent activator of aldehyde dehydrogenase, and therefore, its supplementation appears to reduce acetaldehyde concentration following ingestion of ethanol [38].

Tryptophan

Alcoholics have elevated tryptophan levels in the cerebrospinal fluid compared with healthy controls; they also have decreased plasma levels of this amino acid. This remains unchanged even after abstention from ethanol in patients with alcoholic liver disease [47].

There is a decreased ratio of tryptophan to other amino acids competing for brain transport, which may be associated with depression [48], suicidal ideation [49], aggression [50], memory impairment and blackouts [51], as well as with convulsions [52].

Effects of ethanol on digestion and use of other nutrients

β-Carotene

Alcoholic patients tend to have low plasma carotene levels presumably due to its low intake, ethanol itself may, in fact, increase β-carotene blood levels, due to a possible blockage in the conversion of β-carotene to retinol (vitamin A) by ethanol [53,65].

Carnitine

Carnitine appears to inhibit alcohol-induced fatty liver by facilitating the oxidation of the increased fatty acid load produced by alcohol ingestion [54].

Choline

A deficiency of choline has provided a mechanism for studies duplicating the morphologic changes encountered in human subjects who inject alcohol. Mice, rats, rabbits, dogs, monkeys, and humans put on a choline deficient diet develop fatty liver, fibrosis, and cirrhosis. Studies of choline deficient animals have clarified the morphologic and biochemical changes seen in the alcoholic. Choline has been useful in eliminating fatty liver of the diabetic, alcoholic, and other conditions, which produce liver dysfunction.

Glutathione

Glutathione plays a dual role: on one hand, it protects the liver from alcohol-induced damage; on the other, it protects the gastric mucosa from alcohol-induced damage [55].

Lecithin (phosphatidyl choline)

A significant decrease of liver phpholipids in general and of phosphatidyl choline in particular is associated with chronic alcohol consumption. Administering polyunsaturated lecithin may correct these deficiencies, and may prevent alcohol-induced fibrosis and cirrhosis [56].

Omega 6 fatty acids

Ethanol blocks the conversion of linoleic acid to gamma linoleic acid, and increases the conversion of dihommogamma linoleic acid to prostaglandin E1, resulting in a gamma linoleic acid deficiency. Its supplementation may at least theoretically prevent alcohol toxicity [20,57] and reduce the severity of alcohol withdraw [20,58].

Supplementation with essential fatty acids may promote recovery of brain function in abstinent alcoholics [59,60].

Panthetine

Panthetine is a derivate of panthothenic and a precursor of coenzyme A. Supplementation with panthetine may reduce the adverse effects caused by accumulation of acetaldehyde by increasing the activity of acetaldehyde dehydrogenase [33,61].

Homocysteine

Homocysteine plasma levels are elevated among alcoholics. In a clinical study, 42 alcoholic patients were hospitalized for detoxification. These subjects had significantly higher homocysteine levels compared with controls on admission. Two weeks later, the same group of patients had normal concentrations of homocysteine in plasma [62]. The same authors suggested that there might be a correlation between high homocysteine levels and increased incidence of stroke in alcoholics.

Caffeine

Although heavy coffee consumption may stimulate ethanol craving in alcoholics, small amounts of caffeine appear to protect the liver from adverse effects of alcohol [20]. It has been reported that there are lower levels of gamma glutamil transferase, which is usually elevated in alcoholic liver disease, among coffee drinkers compared with controls [63].

Summary

Liver disease of the alcoholic is associated with a significant alteration of other body systems because of the influence of ethanol on the body's nutrient balance (i.e. vitamins, minerals, and amino acids). The most prominent clinical alteration results from changes in vitamin nutriture, deficits of the thiamine leading to Wernicke's encephalopathy and peripheral neuropathy, depletion of niacin evoking pellagra, pyridoxamine loss causing neurological dysfunction, and deficits of vitamin B12 and folic acid evoking central nervous system medicated impairment. In the absence of specific knowledge of the presence or absence of a deficiency state contributing to liver failure in alcoholic liver disease, the supplemental treatment for a possible B12 and folate deficiency is desirable in the absence of skin or neurological alterations.

Each of the nutrient deficit groups exhibit increase in morbidity and mortality form alcoholic liver disease. Corrective therapy designed to eliminate the causative factors is often life saving. A most dramatic response is noted in treatment of B12 and/or folate deficits associated with alcoholic hepatitis. Since the nutrients play a central role in protecting uninjured liver cells and stimulation repair or replacement of damaged cells, their replacement with deficient, is essential and often life saving. Artificaial assists are useful in eliminating endogenous and exogenous substances, which cannot be removed by the sick liver. Correction of a deficiency of nucleic acid precursors and catalysts of suppression of circulatory antagonist, which interfere with cell replication, may facilitate production of new hepatocytes inpatients with reversible injury or DNA and RNA templates [14].

References

[1] Ward RJ, Petters TJ. The antioxidant status of patients with either alcohol induced liver damage or myopathy. Alcohol 1992;27:359–65.

[2] Majumdar SK, Thompson AD, et al. Vitamin A utilization status in chronic alcoholic patients. Int J Vitam Nutr Res 1983;53(3):273–9.

[3] Marotta F, Labadarios D, Frazer L, et al. Fat soluble vitamin concentration in chronic alcohol induced pancreatitis. Dig Dis Sci 1994;39:369–71.

[4] Avila MA, Carretero V, Rodriguez N, et al. Regulation by hypoxia of methionine adenosyl transferase activity and gene expression in rat hepatocytes. Gastroenterology 1998;114:369–71.

[5] Thompson AD, Majumdar SK. The Influence of ethanol on intestinal absorption and utilization of nutrients. Gastroenterology 1981;10:263–93.

[6] Scholmerich J, Lohla E, Gerok W, et al. Zinc and vitamin A deficiency in liver cirrhosis. Hepatogastroenterology 1982;30:1333–8.

[7] Lieber CS. Biochemical and molecular basis of alcohol-induced injury to liver and other tissues. N Engl J Med 1988;319(25):1639–50.

[8] Leo MA, Lieber CS. Hepatic vitamin A depletion in alcoholic liver injury. N Engl J Med 1982;307:562–72.

[9] Leo MA, Lieber CS. Hepatic fibrosis after long term administration of ethanol and moderate vitamin A supplementation in the rat. Hepatology 1983;3:1–11.

[10] Leo MA, Loewe N, Lieber CS. Decreased hepatic vitamin A after drug administration in men and in rats. Am J Clin Nutr 1984;40:1131–6.

[11] Leo MA, Lieber CS. Alcohol, vitamin A and beta carotene: adverse interactions, including hepatotoxicity and carcinogenicity. Am J Clin Nutr 1999;69:79–85.

[12] Pollack ES, Nomura A, Heilbrum L, et al. Prospective study of alcohol consumption and cancer. N Engl J Med 1984;310:617–21.

[13] Lieber CS, Leo MA. Potentation of ethanol-induced hepatic vitamin A depletion by pheno-barbital and butylated hydroxitoluene. J Nutr 1984;117:70–6.

[14] Kvale G, Bielke F, Gart JJ. Diet habits and Lung cancer risk. Int J Cancer 1993;31:397–405.

[15] Leevy CM. Thiamin deficiency and alcoholism. Ann NY Acad Sci 1982;378:316–24.

[16] Paladin F, Russo Perez G. The haematic thiamine level in the course of alcoholic neuropathy. Eur Neurol 1987;26(3):129–33.

[17] Leevy CM, Thompson AD, Baker H. Vitamins and liver injury. Am J Clin Nutr 1965;23: 346–61.

[18] Kim C-I, Roe A. Development of riboflavin deficiency in alcohol-fed hamster drug–nutrient interactions. Drug Nutr Interact 1985;3:13.

[19] Ishii N, Nishihara Y. Pellagra among chronic alcoholics: clinical and pathological study of 20 necropsy cases. J Neurol Neurosurg Psychiatry 1981;44:209–15.

[20] Werbach MR. Nutritional influences on illness; a source book for clinical research. 1996. p. 25–92.

[21] Duce AM, Ortiz P, Cabrero C, et al. S-adenosyl-L-methionine synthetase and phospholipid methyltransferase are inhibited in human cirrhosis. Hepatology 1988;8:65–8.

[22] (a) Lumeng L, Li T-K, Bshear RE, et al. Clearance and metabolism of plasma pyridoxal 5′phosphate in the dog. J Lab Clin Med 1978;103:286–93.
    (b) Vech RL, Li TK. Vitamin B6 methabolism in chronic alcohol abuse. J Clin Invest 1975;55: 1026–32.

[23] Fonda ML, Brown SG, Pendelton MW. Concentration of vitamin B6 anactivities of enzymes of B6 metabolism in the blood of alcoholic and nonalcoholic men. Alcohol Clin Exp Res 1989; 3:804.

[24] Lieber CS. Alcohol: its metabolism and interactions with nutrients. Annu Rev Nutr 2000;20: 395–430.

[25] Leevy CM, Baker H. Vitamins and alcoholism. Am J Clin Nutr 1968;16:339–46.

[26] Kanazawa S, Herbert V. Total corrinoid, cobalamin (viamin B12), and cobalamin analogue levels may be normal in serum despite cobalamin's liver depletion in patients with alcoholism. Lab Invest 1985;53:108–10.

[27] McMartin KE, Milikan WJ, McGhee A. Cumulative excess urinary excretion of folate in rats after repeated ethanol treatment. J Nutr 1986;116:1316–25.

[28] Tamura T, Halstead CH. Folate turnover in chronically alcoholic monkeys. J Lab Clin Med 1983;97:654–61.

[29] Bonjour JP. Vitamins and alcoholism II. Int J Vitam Nutr 1980;49:96–121.

[30] DiLuzio NR. A mechanism of the acute ethanol-induced fatty liver and the modification of liver injury by antioxidants. Lab Invest 1966;15:50–61.

[31] Clot P, Tabone M, Arico S, et al. Monitoing oxidating damage in patients with liver cirrhosis and different daily alcohol intake. Gut 1994;35:1637–43.

[32] P'a de la Maza M, Petermann M, Bunout D, et al. Effects of long-term vitamin E sup-plementation in alcoholic cirrhotics. J Am Coll Nutr 1995;14(2):192–6.

[33] Pitts TO, Thiel DH. Disorders of divalent ions and vitamin D metabolism in chronic alcoholism. Recent Dev Alcohol 1986;4:357–77.

[34] Jacques PF, et al. Moderate alcohol intake and nutritional status in nonalcoholic elderly subjects. Am J Clin Nutr 1989;50:875–83.

[35] Savage D, Lindenbaum J. Anemia in alcoholics. Medicine (Baltimore) 1986. p. 322–7.

[36] Barbe B, Lejoyeux M, Bouleau JH, et al. Visual hallucinations related to severe hypophospha-taemia [lLetter]. Lancet 1991;338:1083.

[37] Knochel JP. The pathophysiology and clinical characteristics of severe hypophosphatemia. Arch Intern Med 1977;137:203–20.

[38] Watanabe A, Hubora N, Nagashima H, et al. Lowering of liver acetaldehyde but not ethanol concentrations by pretreatment with taurine in ethanol-loaded rats. Experientia 1985;41(11): 1421–2.

[39] Preedy VR, Marvay JS, McIntosh A, et al. Gastrointestinal protein turnover and alcohol misuse. Drug Alcohol Depend 1993;34:141–67.

[40] Braona E, Leo M, Bowsky SA, et al. Alcoholic hepatomegaly: accumulation of protein in the liver. Science 1975;190:794–5.

[41] Shaw S, Lieber CS. Plasma amino acids in the alcoholic: nutritional aspects. Alcoholism (NY) 1983;7(1):22–7.

[42] Rogers LL, Pelton RB. Glutamine in the treatment of alcoholism. Q J Stud Alcohol 1957;18(4): 581–7.

[43] Blum K, Wallace JE, Friedman RN. Reduction of acute alcohol intoxication by a amino acids: glycine and serine. Life Sci 1974;14:557–65.

[44] Kinsell L, Harper HA, Barton HC, et al. Rate of disappearance from plasma of intravenously administret methionine in patients with liver damage. Science 1947;106:583–94.

[45] Finkelstein JD, Martin JJ. Methionine metabolism in mammals. Adaptation to methionine excess. J Biol Chem 1986;261:1212–5.

[46] Mato JM, Lieber CS, Kaplowitz N, et al, editors. Methionine metabolism: molecular mechanism and clinical implications. Madrid: SA Bouncopy; 1992. p. 1–232.

[47] Beck O, Borg SS, Sedval GG, et al. Tryptophan levels in human cerebrospinal fluid after acute and chronic ehtanol consumption. Drug Alcohol Depend 1983;12(3):217–22.

[48] Branchey L, Branchey MH, Noumair D, et al. Ethanol impairs tryptophan transport into the brain and depresses serotonin. Life Sci 1981;26:2751–5.

[49] Branchey L, Brightwell DR, et al. Relationship between changes in plasma amino acids and depression in alcoholic patients. Am J Psychiatry 1984;141(1):1212–5.

[50] Branchey L, Branchey MH, Noumair D, et al. Depression, suicide and aggression in alcoholics and their relationship to plasma amino acids. Psychiatr Res 1984;12(3):219–26.

[51] Branchey L, Brightwell DR, Derman RM, et al. Association between low plasma tryptophan and blackouts in male alcoholic patients. Alcoholism (NY) 1985;9(5):393–5.

[52] Marion JL, Petit EF, Viltord S, et al. Alcoholic epilepsy. Decrease of tryptophan levels in the blood and cerebrospinal fluid. Presse Med 1985;14(12):681–3.

[53] Leo MA, Kim C, Lowe N, et al. Interaction of ethanol with b-carotene: delayed blood clearance and enhanced hepatotoxicity. Hepatology 1992;15:883–91.

[54] Sachan DL, Rhew TH, Ruark RA. Ameliorating effects of carnitine and its precursors on alcohol-induced fatty liver. Am J Clin Nutr 1984;39:738–44.

[55] Loguercio C, Taranto D, Beneduce F, et al. Glutathione prevents ethanol induced gastric mucosal damage and depletion of sulphhydryl compounds in humans. Gut 1993;34:161–5.

[56] Lieber CS, Li J-J, Robins S, et al. Dietary dilinoleoylphosphatidylcholine (CLPC) is incorporated into liver phospholipids, protects against alcoholic cirrhosis, enhances collaglenase activity and prevents acetaldehyde-ineduced collagen accumulation in cultured lipocytes. Hepatol Abstr 1992;16:87A.

[57] Karpe F, Wejde J, Anggard E, et al. The effect of dietary primrose oil on ethanol withdrawal in the rat. Acta Pharmacol Toxicol 1983;53:16–8.

[58] Horrobin DF. A biochemical basis for alcoholism and alcohol-induced damage including the fetal alcohol syndrome and cirrhosis: interference with essential fatty acid and prostaglandin metabolism. Med Hypotheses 1980;6:929–42.

[59] MacDonnell LDF, Skinner FK, Glen AIM. Effects of essential fatty acid supplementation on neuropsychological function in abstinent alcoholics. In Developments in clinical and experimental neuropsychology. New York: Plenum Press; 1989.

[60] Skinner FK, MacDonnell LEF, Glen EMT, et al. Impairment of alcohol-dependent subjects and change over six months in two double-blind trials using essential fatty acid supplementation. In Proc 35th Int Congress in Alcoholism and Drug Dependence vol. 4. Oslo; 1988. p. 300–8.

[61] Leevy CM, Baker H, et al. B-complex vitamins in liver disease of the alcoholic. Am J Clin Nutr 1965.

[62] Hultberg B, Berglund M, Andersson A, et al. Elevated plasma homocysteine in alcoholics. Alcohol Clin Exp Res 1993;17:687–9.

[63] Kono S, Shinchi K, Imanishi K, et al. Coffee and serum gamma-glutamyltransferase. Am J Epidemiol 1944;139:723–7.

[64] Treloar A, Larner AJ, Crook M, et al. Hypophosphataemia, hallucinations, and delerium tremens [letter]. Lancet 1991;338:1467–8.

[65] Ahmed S, Leo MA, Lieber CS. Interactions between alcohol and b-carotene in patients with alcoholic liver disease. Am J Clin Nutr 1994;60:430–6.

ELSEVIER
SAUNDERS

CLINICS IN
LIVER DISEASE

Clin Liver Dis 9 (2005) 83–101

Effect of Alcohol on Viral Hepatitis and Other Forms of Liver Dysfunction

Sripriya Balasubramanian, MD[a], Kris V. Kowdley, MD[b],*

[a]*Division of Gastroenterology and Hepatology, University of California at Davis,
4150 V Street #3500, Sacramento, California 95817, USA*
[b]*Division of Gastroenterology and Hepatology, University of Washington, Box 356174,
1959 NE Pacific Street, Seattle, Washington 98195, USA*

Alcohol is a known hepatotoxic agent, which may exacerbate liver injury caused by other agents. The wide prevalence of alcohol use and abuse in society makes it an important cofactor in many other liver diseases. Examples of liver diseases that are significantly influenced by ingestion of alcohol include chronic viral hepatitis, disorders of iron overload, and obesity-related liver disease.

The two most common causes of chronic viral hepatitis worldwide are hepatitis B and hepatitis C. Along with alcoholic liver disease, these viruses are responsible for most cases of cirrhosis of the liver end-stage liver disease and hepatocellular cancer (HCC) worldwide. The interaction between alcohol and viral hepatitis in the pathogenesis of liver disease is highly variable in individual patients. In this review, we examine the effect of alcohol on liver disease from viral hepatitis in patients with chronic hepatitis C and hepatitis B, in addition to coinfection of human immunodeficiency virus (HIV) with hepatitis B or C. The role of alcohol in influencing the clinical presentations of hemochromatosis, African iron overload, and underlying mechanisms are discussed. Newer data on

---

K.V.K. was supported by NIH Grants 38215, 02957, and 54698.

S.B. was supported by an AASLD Schering advanced hepatology fellowship training grant.

* Corresponding author.

E-mail address: kkowdley@u.washington.edu (K.V. Kowdley).

the possible effect of alcohol ingestion in small quantities on liver disease related to obesity and the metabolic syndrome are also reviewed.

Hepatitis C

Hepatitis C is the most common liver disease in the United States, with approximately 4 million infected individuals [1]. It has been estimated that about 14 million Americans are estimated to have some form of alcohol dependence [2]. The prevalence of hepatitis C antibody seropositivity among chronic alcoholics worldwide is higher than in the general population, although estimates vary among studies and geographic locations. A confounding factor is that early studies relied on the use of hepatitis C antibody positivity for diagnosis without the concomitant use of polymerase chain reaction (PCR) for confirmation of the presence of hepatitis C RNA and reported prevalence rates of hepatitis C of up to 50% in chronic alcoholics [3]. Worldwide, prevalence rates for hepatitis C in studies incorporating PCR confirmation vary between 11% in Sweden [4] to 44% in Japan [5] among alcoholic patients. In the United States, hepatitis C positivity rates among alcoholics based on studies using hepatitis C virus (HCV) RNA testing vary between 16% to 23% [6,7].

Studies of HCV prevalence that do not specifically focus on alcoholics, such as a study of 1098 veterans receiving medical care in the New York metropolitan area, also demonstrate an independent association of alcohol abuse with HCV seropositivity confirmed by PCR assays [8]. In this study, a history of alcohol abuse conferred almost as high a risk of acquiring HCV infection as prior exposure to blood during combat (odds ratio [OR] 2.4 versus 2.6). The higher prevalence of hepatitis C antibody in chronic alcoholics has been attributed to the coexistence of high-risk behaviors such as injection drug use in this population. However, some data suggest that this higher prevalence may not be attributable to such confounding factors alone. Hepatitis B, also transmitted by similar parenteral routes, is not increased in alcoholics, while prevalence of hepatitis C is increased as much as 20-fold when compared with the general population [9]. This would lead to a hypothesis that alcohol use in some way enhances the acquisition and persistence of HCV upon exposure to the virus, although direct evidence of this is lacking.

Enhanced viral replication of HCV in alcoholics has been observed in a number of studies. Cromie et al [10] demonstrated higher viral titers in patients with hepatitis C who consumed large amounts of alcohol in comparison with abstinent patients. Similarly, in the study by Poynard [11] establishing the accelerated progression of liver disease in patients who consumed in excess of 50 g/d of alcohol, higher levels of viremia were demonstrated in the group with heavy alcohol consumption. Interestingly, a study by Pessione et al [12] demonstrated an independent association between even moderate alcohol consumption (< 140 g of alcohol/wk) and hepatitis C viral load in 233 patients with hepatitis C [12].

Abstinence from alcohol has also been shown to result in a reduction of viremia [10,13,14].

Alcohol use and natural history of hepatitis C

Studies on the effects of alcohol use in the natural history of hepatitis C have mainly focused on the effects of chronic heavy alcohol consumption. Seeff et al [15] found increased mortality related to liver disease in a cohort of patients with non-A non-B hepatitis and heavy alcohol use. Almost 70% of the deaths from end-stage liver disease occurred in the subgroup of patients with associated alcoholism [15]. A number of studies have evaluated the effects of chronic heavy alcohol use on disease progression. In 1997, Poynard et al [11] reported the results of a cross-sectional study evaluating disease progression in a cohort of 1157 French patients with treatment of naïve hepatitis C who had undergone a single liver biopsy. Alcohol use was recorded through a standardized questionnaire, based on the number of drinks per day. Using a multivariate analysis of host and virus-derived risk factors (ie, age at infection, gender, alcohol use, virus genotype, and viral load), the authors demonstrated that alcohol consumption of greater than 50 g/d of alcohol was an independent risk factor for advanced fibrosis (OR 2.36 and 1.49 in the two models of multivariate analysis) (Fig. 1) [11]. The limitations of this study included the use of a single biopsy and an estimated duration of infection to calculate the fibrosis score. This was partially offset by the use for validation of the model in a smaller sample of 70 patients who had undergone paired liver biopsies, without intervening therapy for hepatitis C, and in another subset of patients with transfusion-associated hepatitis C in whom the date of acquisition was known. Observed fibrosis progression scores in these subsets were similar to the calculated fibrosis score in the study cohort [11]. Another cross-sectional study from France, published the same year, included 6664 patients with hepatitis C. Threshold alcohol consumption in this study was six drinks/d for men and five drinks/day for women, above which there was an increased risk of fibrosis progression (34.9% versus 18.2% in non-drinkers) [16]. A similar study of 234 Australian patients with HCV attending a tertiary care clinic found an independent correlation between lifetime alcohol intake and fibrosis score, while mean daily alcohol intake was not predictive of fibrosis stage. This led the authors to conclude that the duration of drinking history was an important determinant of disease progression [13]. Thomas et al [17] found in a longitudinal study of 1667 American HCV-positive patients, many with HIV coinfection, that incidence of end-stage liver disease during a mean follow-up of 8.8 years was higher in patients with heavy alcohol intake defined as greater than 260 g/wk. These authors failed to demonstrate a statistically significant increase in risk with consumption of lower amounts of alcohol. Another retrospective study by Harris et al [18] demonstrated a fourfold increased risk of cirrhosis among patients with hepatitis C who consumed greater than 80 g/d of alcohol.

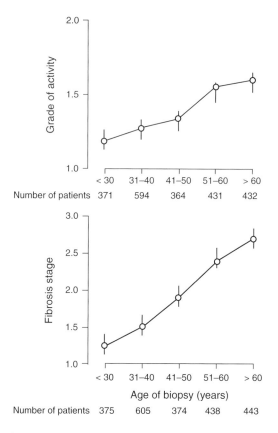

Fig. 1. Association between stage of fibrosis and age at biopsy or duration of infection by alcohol consumption (*From* Poynard T, Bedossa P, Opolon P. Natural history of liver fibrosis progression in patients with chronic hepatitis C. The OBSVIRC, METAVIR, CLINIVIR, and DOSVIRC groups. Lancet 1997;349(9055):825–32, with permission.)

Serfaty et al [19] compared 84 cirrhotic patients with HCV to a matched group of 84 noncirrhotic controls with hepatitis C, drawn from a population of 464 patients hospitalized during the same period. Although no differences were found between the two groups in other factors evaluated such as viral genotype or alpha 1 antitrypsin phenotype, a significant difference was noted in alcohol intake between cirrhotic and noncirrhotic patients. Significantly more alcohol use was noted among cases than controls, particularly in the group that consumed 30 to 80 g/d of alcohol. A trend toward alcohol intake of greater than 80 g/d in cirrhotics was also noted but was not statistically significant. The authors concluded that even moderate alcohol intake (ie, 30–80 g/d) was a risk factor for increased disease progression. A similar case–control study from Italy compared two cohorts of cirrhotics with HCV to a control population of patients admitted to the hospital for other acute problems, including orthopedic surgeries, lifetime daily alcohol intake of 75 to 100 g/d (first cohort), and 125 g/d or greater (second cohort) was synergistic with HCV in the development of fibrosis. No synergism was noted with consumption of alcohol at levels less than 50 g/d [20]. This latter study included the relatively healthy controls for cases with cirrhosis, which may have biased the results toward overestimating the effect of alcohol.

A number of limitations are common to these studies examining the relationship between HCV and alcohol use that involve both study methodology and methods of estimation of alcohol intake. With the exception of the study by Thomas et al [11–13,16,17,19–21], all the other studies involve a cross-sectional methodology where fibrosis scores at a single point in time are used to estimate the effects of long-term and ongoing alcohol use. Methods used to estimate alcohol intake varied between studies. Although all were based on patient recall and self-report, two [16,20] are based on data abstracted from patients' charts, which may be less reliable. Although reports based on self-reporting for alcohol use may also be flawed, such studies use standardized questionnaires, sometimes repeated over multiple time points, and in addition, may include the computation of a lifetime daily alcohol intake [17,22,23] to minimize errors in estimation. Despite these methodologic concerns, there is agreement among studies that heavy alcohol use in hepatitis C is detrimental. There appears to be a consensus that long-term heavy alcohol use accelerates progression of disease in chronic hepatitis C.

The use of occasional or small amounts of alcohol is a much more controversial issue. This is an important question, however, because alcohol is purported to have benefits in terms of reducing insulin resistance and to have antioxidant effects [24,25]; thus, patients with hepatitis C may potentially be advised to drink red wine by their cardiologists to reduce their cardiovascular risk. Most previous studies were not designed with the intent to elicit data on patients who were using small quantities of alcohol. In fact, there are conflicting results among studies that primarily addressed populations where mean alcohol intake was moderate or low. A study by Pessione et al [12] reported a strong correlation between past alcohol intake (ie, before diagnosis of HCV) and fibrosis stage in a cross-sectional study involving 233 patients. This effect was demonstrated in a population where the majority of subjects (88%) consumed less than 210 g/wk of alcohol (less than three drinks/d), leading the authors to conclude that even moderate consumption enhanced fibrogenesis [12]. One of the problems with this study is that estimation of past alcohol intake was elicited solely by the amount of alcohol consumed in the week before diagnosis of HCV infection, which may be less accurate than other methods such as the computation of lifetime daily alcohol intake. Another study by Westin et al [22] involved 78 Swedish patients with hepatitis C, all of whom had paired biopsies to assess fibrosis progression. Alcohol intake was quantified for all patients as cumulative intake, taking periods of abstinence into account. Median alcohol consumption for this group was 4.8 g/d. Patients who had consumed more than a cumulative amount of 8600 g of alcohol had worse fibrosis than those who consumed less, but the time between biopsies in the two groups differed by almost a year. The authors state that this difference was statistically insignificant; yet, the time between biopsies was an independent predictor of fibrosis stage on multivariate analysis. Drinking frequency but not quantity of alcohol consumed was correlated with fibrosis progression in multi-variate analysis. Another study by Cholet et al [26], in a sample of patients that consumed little or no alcohol, wherein only 15% of the cohort consumed greater than 80 g/d of alcohol, found advanced fibrosis to be significantly associated with all levels of alcohol intake greater than 20 g/d on univariate analysis; how-ever, alcohol intake at any level was not independently predictive of fibrosis in multivariate analysis. The Trent HCV study group [27] prospectively evaluated 214 patients with repeat biopsies, spaced a mean of 2.5 years apart, and found no correlation between alcohol intake and fibrosis progression. Alcohol intake in this group has not been reported, apart from being quantified as "low." In a recent cross-sectional study of alcohol use in 800 patients with hepatitis C, Monto et al [23] have demonstrated no association between light and moderate alcohol intake, defined as less than 50 g/d of alcohol, and fibrosis progression. Yet, the authors noted that when the cohort was divided into quintiles based on quantity of alcohol consumed, there was a stepwise increase in mean fibrosis score with increasing alcohol use.

Another factor complicating the study of alcohol consumption and disease severity in HCV is the possibility that insulin resistance may be a consequence of chronic HCV infection [28], and may contribute to hepatic fibrogenesis [29]. Successful treatment with interferon is associated with improvement in insulin sensitivity [30]. Because there are also data linking improvement in insulin sen-sitivity to moderate alcohol use [24,25], additional studies examining the effect of mild to moderate alcohol consumption in patients with HCV are warranted.

Effects of excessive alcohol consumption on the liver in viral hepatitis have been studied in humans as well as animal models. There are data to suggest that alcohol may exert synergistic effects on liver injury from viral hepatitis through effects on viral replication [31], alteration of immune responses, promotion of hepatic iron deposition, and impaired liver regeneration [32]. In addition, in an Australian study that examined liver biopsies from patients with HCV who also completed a questionnaire detailing lifetime daily alcohol intake, alcohol was shown to augment HCV-induced hepatocyte apoptosis as detected by in situ terminal nick end uridine triphosphate (UTP) (part of TUNEL, terminal uridine triphosphate nick end labelling) labeling. Fas expression was also increased in patients with HCV who consumed any alcohol in comparison with abstinent patients, leading to the inference that alcohol increases virus-induced hepatocyte apoptosis in patients with HCV by Fas-dependent mechanisms [33]. Alcohol has also been demonstrated to induce hepatocyte apoptosis by Fas-independent mechanisms, such as glutathione depletion, which sensitizes hepatocytes to the action of tumor necrosis factor-alpha, in alcohol-fed rats [34]. It is thus hypothe-sized that the observed increase in hepatocyte apoptosis in chronic hepatitis C may occur through both Fas-dependent and -independent mechanisms [33]. This finding of increased apoptosis is important in light of new evidence linking hepatocyte apoptosis to fibrogenesis. Kupffer cell engulfment of apoptotic bodies has been demonstrated to result in a profibrogenic response in a bile duct ligated mouse model [35]. Engulfment of apoptotic bodies by stellate cells is shown in human immortalized stellate cell lines to result in activation and production of collagen [36]. Activated stellate cells are the primary effectors of hepatic fibrogenesis [37]; this may explain in part clinical observations of accelerated fibrosis in viral hepatitis with concomitant heavy alcohol use. Other well-recognized profibrogenic factors include hepatic iron deposition, which occurs as a result of chronic alcohol use and potentiates liver damage from viral injury through the generation of reactive oxygen species and oxidative stress [38]. Oxidative stress is a potent stimulus for stellate cell activation and collagen deposition, also resulting in increased fibrosis [38].

Immune responses are globally altered in chronic alcoholics, and include effects primarily on innate immune responses [39]. The exact mechanism of the interaction between HCV viral proteins and the innate immune system is not well understood, and little is known about the effect of alcohol on this interaction. Studies in acute hepatitis C have demonstrated that a broad and vigorous T-cell response is important for clearance of acute infection in both humans [40,41] and in chimpanzees [42]. T-cell function is demonstrated to be impaired in chronic alcoholics [43,44]. Another study of human volunteers fed 0.8 mg/kg body weight of alcohol (equivalent to about three drinks/d) demonstrated reduction in T-cell function, as well as accessory cell function, associated with reduced production of interferon gamma and elevated levels of IL 10 and IL 13 within 18 hours of ingestion [45]. This study addresses effects of acute alcohol ingestion on immunity; however, other mechanisms may be important in chronic alcoholics. The changes described with alcohol are also indicative of favoring the Th2 subtype immune response, which is associated with persistence of infection [40,46]. Dendritic cells, which are antigen-presenting cells and allostimulatory to T cells, are important in clearance of hepatitis C [47]. Impaired function of dendritic cells has been reported in patients with chronic hepatitis C [48]; alcohol has also been shown in healthy volunteers to reduce dendritic cell maturation independently and in concert with HCV in patients with chronic hepatitis, through a reduced production of IL-2 [49]. Encke et al [50] studied the response to a HCV nonstructural protein NS5, recognized as important for viral clearance, in an ethanol-fed mouse model. They found significant impairment of B-cell, T-helper cell, and cytotoxic T-cell function. Although B-cell and T-helper cell function showed some improvement with abstinence, cytotoxic T-cell functional impairment remained unchanged. In summary, indirect evidence indicates that alcohol has effects on suppression of T-cell function, which may contribute to persistence of HCV infection upon exposure to virus. Studies designed to address the effect of alcohol on HCV-specific immunity in chronic hepatitis are warranted to further clarify the role of alcohol induced immune suppression in hepatitis C.

Effect of alcohol on therapy of hepatitis C

Alcohol abuse has long been considered a contraindication to therapy of hepatitis C with interferon-based therapy, primarily because of concerns regarding compliance to interferon-based therapy in patients with a history of substance abuse [51]. Furthermore, there are data to indicate that alcohol may have other effects on response to therapy, which are independent of compliance effects. Response rates to interferon therapy are lowered by alcohol use, and the magnitude of the effect increases with increasing alcohol use [52–54]. An Italian study of patients with hepatitis C and history of alcohol use, undergoing Interferon therapy after 6 months of abstinence, showed that the sustained response rate felt from 33% in nondrinkers to 20% of mild drinkers (23–69 g/d of alcohol) and to only 9% in heavy drinkers (>69 g/d of alcohol). Abstinence during therapy was confirmed by carbohyderate-deficient transferrin measurement. Relapse rates after treatment were increased twofold in past consumers of any amount of alcohol when compared with nondrinkers [54]. Postulated mechanisms for a reduced response to therapy involve higher viral replication in alcoholics [10], higher viral load [10,12,14], depressive effects of alcohol on cell-mediated immunity [43], and in addition, increased viral quasi-species complexity in alcoholics [55].

Effect of alcohol on hepatitis B

Hepatitis B virus (HBV) affects more than 350 million individuals worldwide [56], and approximately 1.25 million individuals in the United States are chronic carriers of HBV [57]. Alcohol has been shown to enhance hepatitis B viral replication in transgenic mice [58]. A study of 1113 Japanese patients with chronic hepatitis B revealed that Hepatitis B e antigen prevalence tends to be higher and decrease more slowly with age in heavy drinkers (defined as greater than 60 g/d of alcohol) than in nondrinkers, suggesting that alcohol abuse may delay Hepatitis B e antigen loss [59]. Effects of alcohol on progression of fibrosis in chronic hepatitis B have not been examined in detail; the current evidence suggests that alcohol use is associated with increased risk of cirrhosis and HCC in chronic HBV infection [60,61]. In studies of patients who were hepatitis B surface antigen positive, alcohol intake of more than 60 g/d of ethanol was associated with increased necroinflammatory changes on liver biopsy [62] as well as serum liver biochemical test abnormalities [63].

Effect of alcohol on hepatocellular cancer

HCC develops in patients with chronic liver disease irrespective of etiology of the liver disease, although the incidence is relatively high in viral hepatitis [64]. Data from several studies strongly suggest that heavy alcohol use is a significant additive risk in hepatocarcinogenesis in the setting of chronic viral hepatitis, especially among smokers [65] and those with noninsulin-dependent diabetes mellitus [66]. Alcohol intake of greater than 60 g/d is associated with a twofold increase in HCC in viral hepatitis [67]. A recent large population-based cohort study of over 11,000 men in Taiwan found that alcohol use, in addition to smoking and betel quid chewing (a practice of chewing two halves of an areca nut, sandwiched between a betel leaf that is coated with red slaked lime [68]), significantly increased risk of HCC in both HBs Ag-positive and -negative individuals, and the highest adjusted risk ratio was in HBs Ag-positive individuals with substance abuse defined by smoking, betel quid chewing, and alcohol use [69].

Effect of alcohol on viral hepatitis coinfected with human immunodeficiency virus

Hepatitis B, C, and HIV share common parenteral routes of transmission, and all three viruses may coexist in the same patient. Thomas et al [17], in their prospective study of patients with chronic hepatitis C, found that patients coinfected with HIV were less likely to spontaneously clear hepatitis C. Fibrosis progression is accelerated in patients coinfected with HIV and HCV; this effect is further amplified by chronic heavy alcohol use [70–73]. A study of 914 patients who had HIV and HCV coinfection who underwent liver biopsies for abnormal liver function tests found that alcohol intake of greater than 50 g/d was associated with severe liver fibrosis [71]. A similar association between advanced fibrosis and alcohol use has been reported by Tural et al [72], who, in addition, noted that duration of HAART therapy (>6 months) may be protective. Liver fibrosis has also been positively associated with alcohol use of greater than 50 g/d and inversely with the use of protease inhibitor containing HAART therapy and the maintenance of a CD4 count greater than 200/dL [73]. It has also been suggested that alcohol potentiates hepatotoxicity from highly active antiretroviral therapy (HAART) and increases risk of such toxicity by 2- to 10-fold [74]. A Spanish study of patients treated with efavirenz or nevirapine demonstrated that both alcohol use and HCV infection were independent predictors of hepatotoxicity from these drugs [75].

A French nationwide study on mortality in HIV 5 years after the introduction of HAART found that end-stage liver disease accounted for 28% of non–AIDS-related deaths, up significantly since 1997, with hepatitis C implicated in 95% of cases of end stage liver disease (ESLD). Alcohol use was also noted to increase during the same period in this cohort [76]. In the post-HAART era, with improved outcomes from HIV infection, liver disease has become a major cause of mortality, and consumption of alcohol has been implicated in this trend [76,77].

Effect of alcohol on hemochromatosis and other non-HFE- related iron overload syndromes

Hepatic iron deposition and alcohol use have been linked since the initial observation by Gilbert and Grenet [78], in 1896, that the two are commonly associated. Hereditary hemochromatosis is a genetic disorder of iron metabolism, which in most cases is a homozygous Cys282Tyr mutation in the HFE gene. Among patients who express the phenotype of Hereditary Hemochromatosis (HH), chronic hyperabsorption of iron from a normal diet leads to deposition of iron in the parenchyma of multiple organs and can result in cirrhosis, HCC, cardiomyopathy, and diabetes mellitus [79]. Before the discovery of the HFE gene and the C282Y mutation, it was sometimes difficult to distinguish between hereditary hemochromatosis and hepatic iron overload due to alcoholism, because heavy alcohol use is associated with increased body iron stores [79]. The hepatic iron index was introduced as a means of differentiating hepatic iron overload from iron overload due to hemochromatosis by introducing an age correction to the hepatic iron concentration [80].

The link between alcohol use and iron overload in the liver has been the focus of several studies. Alcohol is a major regulator of ferritin, inducing its production independent of iron status [81]. Alcoholics have been demonstrated to have upregulation of the transferrin receptor on hepatocytes, which is related to iron uptake [82]. Oxidation of alcohol has been demonstrated to promote dissociation of iron from ferritin, increasing both tissue and serum iron levels [83]. Alcohol and iron are both pro-oxidant stimuli in the liver, and cause hepatotoxicity through mitochondrial injury, upregulation of CYP2E1, depletion of glutathione stores, and the generation of reactive aldehyde products within hepatocytes. These aldehyde products are directly hepatotoxic; they also form protein adducts within the hepatocyte that are immunogenic [84–86]. In addition, oxidative stress results in the activation of hepatic stellate cells, collagen deposition, and hepatic fibrosis [87,88].

The role of alcohol in augmenting the hepatotoxic effects of preexisting iron in the liver has been well studied. Data suggest that free iron in the liver may contribute to hepatic fibrogenesis independent of oxidative stress and exacerbate hepatotoxicity from alcohol [89]. Although iron significantly increases lipid peroxidation in chronically ethanol fed rats [90], the converse, that is, increased lipid peroxidation induced with ethanol feeding in iron-overloaded rats, has not been demonstrated. Experiments of ethanol feeding in rats with iron overload from birth also did not show a significant potentiation of iron-induced hepatic fibrosis by ethanol, although increased hepatocellular injury was demonstrated [91,92].

Several human studies have clearly demonstrated that alcohol use is associated with more severe phenotypic expression and liver disease among patients with hereditary hemochromatosis. Fletcher et al [93], in a study of 202 subjects homozygous for the HFE mutation, demonstrated a ninefold increased risk of cirrhosis in who drank more than 60 g/d of alcohol when compared with individuals who consumed less than 60 g/d (Fig. 2). An earlier study by Adams and Agnew [94], in 1996, retrospectively reviewed clinical features, iron status, alcohol history, liver histology, and long-term survival in 105 putative homozygotes based on HLA identity to a proband with hemochromatosis. Alcohol use of greater than 80 g/d was associated with the presence of cirrhosis and lower

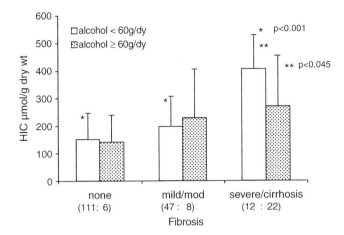

Fig. 2. Relationship between HIC (mean ± SD) and fibrosis in those subjects who consume less than 60 g/d of alcohol (open columns) compared with those who drink greater than or equal to 60 g/d (speckled columns). Numbers in parentheses represent numbers of subjects in each group. *P value between groups with no fibrosis versus severe/cirrhosis; mild/mod fibrosis versus severe/cirrhosis in subjects with alcohol consumption <60 g/d (open columns). **P value comparing patients with severe fibrosis/cirrhosis who consume <60 g/d and those with severe fibrosis/cirrhosis who consume ≥60 g/d. (*From* Fletcher LM, Dixon JL, Purdie DM, Powell LW, Crawford DH. Excess alcohol greatly increases the prevalence of cirrhosis in hereditary hemochromatosis. Gastroenterology 2002; 122(2):281–9, with permission.)

survival, despite the absence of histologic features of alcoholic liver disease on liver biopsy. Another retrospective study from Brittany, France, assessed the effect of alcohol consumption in a cohort of 378 patients with C282Y homozygous hemochromatosis through a self-reported questionnaire. The prevalence of heavy alcohol use in this population was 8.7%, considerably less than that reported in earlier studies. Alcohol consumption of greater than 80 g/d was associated with more severe disease, characterized by higher prevalence of skin pigmentation, diabetes, and hepatomegaly [95]. Available data indicate that alcohol use must be restricted in patients with hereditary hemochromatosis, as it significantly influences the phenotypic expression and severity of disease.

Other iron over load syndromes associated with alcohol use

African iron overload

A syndrome of hepatic iron overload has been described in inhabitants of sub-Saharan or Central Africa, which is associated with the consumption of a tradition alcoholic beverage brewed in iron containers [96]. Initially considered solely a disease of dietary or alcohol induced iron overload, it is now recognized to be associated with a non-HLA-associated genetic defect based on pedigree analysis of affected individuals [97]. Recently, mutations in the ferroportin 1 gene have been described in Africans and in African Americans, associated with mild anemia and a tendency to iron loading [98].

Iron is noted in both parenchymal cells and macrophages, in contrast to hereditary hemochromatosis where iron loading occurs mainly in hepatocytes. High dietary iron content and alcohol use have both been recognized as risk factors for disease. Despite the implication of alcohol in the etiopathogeneis of this disease, histologic features of alcoholic liver disease are usually absent [96]. African iron overload is associated with the development of HCC [99], and is also recognized as a risk factor for death from tuberculosis, which is widely prevalent in the region [100].

Effect of alcohol on liver disease associated with obesity and the metabolic syndrome

Nonalcoholic fatty liver disease (NAFLD) is increasingly recognized as a complication of obesity and insulin resistance syndrome. The metabolic syndrome is characterized by the pentad of insulin resistance, central or visceral obesity, dyslipidemia, impaired glucose tolerance, and hypertension [101]. NAFLD is the form of liver disease characterized by the deposition of fat in the liver that is most commonly seen with obesity, diabetes mellitus, or the metabolic syndrome [102].

Because NAFLD is histologically similar to alcoholic liver disease, it was defined by the exclusion of significant alcohol intake [103,104]. Most early studies describing NAFLD often excluded all patients who consumed any alcohol whatsoever [105]. Later studies did include patients with some alcohol intake; however, there is no clear consensus as to the amount of alcohol that would classify the patient as having "alcoholic" versus "nonalcoholic" liver disease, as evidenced by varying thresholds of alcohol consumption allowed [106,107]. These factors make it is difficult to assess the cumulative or additive effect of light to moderate alcohol consumption in patients who appear to have fatty liver in the setting of obesity and/or insulin resistance. However, there are several published studies that have examined the effects of interaction of obesity and alcohol intake on liver disease outcomes. These are reviewed below.

Low to moderate alcohol intake is shown to improve insulin sensitivity in both normal subjects and those with features of the metabolic syndrome [24,25, 108,109]. This would suggest that mild to moderate alcohol consumption may improve fatty liver by improving insulin resistance. Dixon et al [110] found that moderate alcohol intake in severely obese patients appears to reduce the risk of steatosis, non alcoholic steatohepatitis (NASH), and Mallory bodies seen on liver biopsy, and concluded that moderate alcohol consumption seems to reduce the risk of NAFLD in the severely obese, possibly by reducing insulin resistance. In contrast, another study by Laine et al [111] prospectively evaluated hepatic fibrosis in the metabolic syndrome independent of alcohol consumption, in a population of 173 French patients, and found that total alcohol intake and lifetime mean daily alcohol intake were significantly higher in patients with advanced (F2–F4) fibrosis than those with minimal fibrosis (F0, F1). Ioannou and colleagues [112] studied the effect of obesity on cirrhosis-related death or hospitalization in 11,465 individuals over a mean follow-up period of 12.9 years. Obese individuals were found to be more likely to develop cirrhosis-related death or hospitalization; however, this association was weaker in obese individuals who consumed less than 0.3 alcoholic drinks/d and absent in obese individuals that consumed more than 0.3 alcoholic drinks/d. This is an intriguing finding that may be explained in one of two ways, relating to either the insulin sensitizing or hepatotoxic effects of alcohol consumption. It may be argued that alcohol is protective in obesity-related disease, leading subjects with any alcohol consumption to experience reduced risk of cirrhosis related to NAFLD; alternatively, alcohol consumption in the population may increase the risk of alcoholic cirrhosis, causing it to be equal to the risk of cirrhosis in obesity (Fig. 3).

These conflicting results may be explained in part by the finding that in patients with alcoholic liver disease, body mass index, Perls grade, and blood glucose are independent risk factors for fibrosis [112]. With the current epidemic

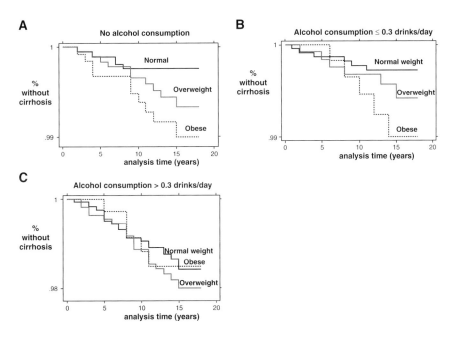

Fig. 3. Kaplan-Meier survival estimates by body mass index category presented separately for participants with (*A*) no alcohol consumption, (*B*) alcohol consumption < 0.3 drinks/d, and (*C*) alcohol consumption >0.3 drinks/d. (*From* Ioannou GN, Weiss NS, Kowdley KV, Dominitz JA. Is obesity a risk factor for cirrhosis-related death or hospitalization? A population-based cohort study. Gastroenterology 2003;125(4):1053–9, with permission.)

of obesity in the United States it is likely that metabolic syndrome-related liver disease will be a significant problem in the future. Clinicians are likely to be confronted with the problems of metabolic syndrome-related liver disease more often. Additional research in this area aimed at further examining the role of mild to moderate alcohol consumption on obesity-related liver disease are warranted, particularly given conflicting recommendations patients receive regarding the risks and benefits of alcohol intake.

References

[1] Kim WR. The burden of hepatitis C in the United States. Hepatology 2002;36(5 Suppl 1): S30–4.

[2] Grant BF. Alcohol consumption, alcohol abuse and alcohol dependence. The United States as an example. Addiction 1994;89(11):1357–65.

[3] Mendenhall CL, Moritz T, Rouster S, et al. Epidemiology of hepatitis C among veterans with alcoholic liver disease. The VA Cooperative Study Group. Am J Gastroenterol 1993;88(7): 1022–6.

[4] Befrits R, Hedman M, Blomquist L, et al. Chronic hepatitis C in alcoholic patients: prevalence, genotypes, and correlation to liver disease. Scand J Gastroenterol 1995;30(11):1113–8.

[5] Shimizu S, Kiyosawa K, Sodeyama T, et al. High prevalence of antibody to hepatitis C virus in heavy drinkers with chronic liver diseases in Japan. J Gastroenterol Hepatol 1992;7(1):30–5.

[6] Coelho-Little ME, Jeffers LJ, Bernstein DE, et al. Hepatitis C virus in alcoholic patients with and without clinically apparent liver disease. Alcohol Clin Exp Res 1995;19(5):1173–6.

[7] Caldwell SH, Li X, Rourk RM, et al. Hepatitis C infection by polymerase chain reaction in alcoholics: false-positive ELISA results and the influence of infection on a clinical prognostic score. Am J Gastroenterol 1993;88(7):1016–21.

[8] Austin GE, Jensen B, Leete J, et al. Prevalence of hepatitis C virus seropositivity among hospitalized US veterans. Am J Med Sci 2000;319(6):353–9.

[9] Rosman AS, Waraich A, Galvin K, et al. Alcoholism is associated with hepatitis C but not hepatitis B in an urban population. Am J Gastroenterol 1996;91(3):498–505.

[10] Cromie SL, Jenkins PJ, Bowden DS, et al. Chronic hepatitis C: effect of alcohol on hepatitic activity and viral titer. J Hepatol 1996;25:821–6.

[11] Poynard T, Bedossa P, Opolon P. Natural history of liver fibrosis progression in patients with chronic hepatitis C. The OBSVIRC, METAVIR, CLINIVIR, and DOSVIRC groups. Lancet 1997;349(9055):825–32.

[12] Pessione F, Degos F, Marcellin P, et al. Effect of alcohol consumption on serum hepatitis C virus RNA and histologic lesions in chronic hepatitis C. Hepatology 1998;27:1717–22.

[13] Ostapowicz G, Watson KJ, Locarnini SA, et al. Role of alcohol in the progression of liver disease caused by hepatitis C virus infection. Hepatology 1998;27(6):1730–5.

[14] Sata M, Fukuizumi K, Uchimura Y. Hepatitis C virus infection in patients with clinically diagnosed alcoholic liver diseases. J Viral Hepat 1996;3(3):143–8.

[15] Seeff LB, Buskell-Bales Z, Wright EC, et al. Long-term mortality after transfusion-associated non-A, non-B hepatitis. The National Heart, Lung, and Blood Institute Study Group. N Engl J Med 1992;327(27):1906–11.

[16] Roudot-Thoraval F, Bastie A, Pawlotsky J-M, et al. Epidemiological factors affecting the severity of hepatitis C virus-related liver disease: a French survey of 6,664 patients. Hepatology 1997;26:485–90.

[17] Thomas DL, Astemborski J, Rai RM, et al. The natural history of hepatitis C virus infection: host, viral, and environmental factors. JAMA 2000;284:450–6.

[18] Harris DR, Gonin R, Alter HJ, et al. The relationship of acute transfusion-associated hepatitis

to the development of cirrhosis in the presence of alcohol abuse. Ann Intern Med 2001;134: 120–4.

[19] Serfaty L, Chazouilleres O, Poujol-Robert A, et al. Risk factors for cirrhosis in patients with chronic hepatitis C virus infection:results of a case–control study. Hepatology 1997;26(3): 776–9.

[20] Corrao G, Arico S. Independent and combined action of hepatitis C virus infection and alcohol consumption on the risk of symptomatic liver cirrhosis. Hepatology 1998;27:914–9.

[21] Poynard T, Ratziu V, Charlotte F, et al. Rates and risk factors of liver fibrosis progression in patients with chronic hepatitis C. J Hepatology 2001;34:730–9.

[22] Westin J, Lagging M, Spak F, et al. Moderate alcohol intake increases fibrosis progression in untreated patients with hepatitis C virus infection. J Viral Hepat 2002;9:235–41.

[23] Monto A, Patel K, Bostrom A, et al. Risks of a range of alcohol intake on hepatitis C-related fibrosis. Hepatology 2004;39(3):826–34.

[24] Goude D, Fagerberg B, Hulthe J, and on behalf of the AIR study group. Alcohol consumption, the metabolic syndrome and insulin resistance in 58-year-old clinically healthy men (AIR study). Clin Sci 2002;102:345–52.

[25] Kiechl S, Willeit J, Poewe W, et al. Insulin sensitivity and regular alcohol consumption: large, prospective, cross sectional population study (Bruneck study). BMJ 1996;313:1040–4.

[26] Cholet F, Nousbaum JB, Richecoeur M, et al. Factors associated with liver steatosis and fibrosis in chronic hepatitis C patients. Gastroenterol Clin Biol 2004;28(3):272–8.

[27] Ryder SD, Irving WL, Jones DA, et al. Trent Hepatitis C Study Group. Progression of hepatic fibrosis in patients with hepatitis C: a prospective repeat liver biopsy study. Gut 2004;53(3): 451–5.

[28] Shintani Y, Fujie H, Miyoshi H, et al. Hepatitis C virus infection and diabetes: direct involvement of the virus in the development of insulin resistance. Gastroenterology 2004;126(3): 840–8.

[29] Sud A, Hui JM, Farrell GC, et al. Improved prediction of fibrosis in chronic hepatitis C using measures of insulin resistance in a probability index. Hepatology 2004;39(5):1239–47.

[30] Konrad T, Vicini P, Zeuzem S, et al. Interferon-alpha improves glucose tolerance in diabetic and non-diabetic patients with HCV-induced liver disease. Exp Clin Endocrinol Diabetes 1999; 107(6):343–9.

[31] Zhang T, Li Y, Lai JP, et al. Alcohol potentiates hepatitis C virus replicon expression. Hepatology 2003;38(1):57–65.

[32] Gao B. Interaction of alcohol and hepatitis viral proteins: implication in synergistic effect of alcohol drinking and viral hepatitis on liver injury. Alcohol 2002;27(1):69–72.

[33] Pianko S, Patella S, Ostapowicz G, et al. Fas-mediated hepatocyte apoptosis is increased by hepatitis C virus infection and alcohol consumption, and may be associated with hepatic fibrosis: mechanisms of liver cell injury in chronic hepatitis C virus infection. J Viral Hepat 2001;8(6):406–13.

[34] Colell A, Garcia-Ruiz C, Miranda M, et al. Selective glutathione depletion of mitochondria by ethanol sensitizes hepatocytes to tumor necrosis factor. Gastroenterology 1998;115(6): 1541–51.

[35] Canbay A, Taimr P, Torok N, et al. Apoptotic body engulfment by a human stellate cell line is profibrogenic. Lab Invest 2003;83(5):655–63.

[36] Canbay A, Feldstein AE, Higuchi H, et al. Kupffer cell engulfment of apoptotic bodies stimulates death ligand and cytokine expression. Hepatology 2003;38(5):1188–98.

[37] Friedman SL. Stellate cell activation in alcoholic fibrosis–an overview. Alcohol Clin Exp Res 1999;23(5):904–10.

[38] Cederbaum AI. Iron and CYP2E1-dependent oxidative stress and toxicity. Alcohol 2003; 30(2):115–20.

[39] Zamara E, Novo E, Marra F, et al. 4-Hydroxynonenal as a selective pro-fibrogenic stimulus for activated human hepatic stellate cells. J Hepatol 2004;40(1):60–8.

[40] Chang KM. Immunopathogenesis of hepatitis C virus infection. Clin Liver Dis 2003;7(1): 89–105.

[41] Ulsenheimer A, Gerlach JT, Gruener NH, et al. Detection of functionally altered hepatitis C virus-specific CD4 T cells in acute and chronic hepatitis C. Hepatology 2003;37(5):1189–98.

[42] Nascimbeni M, Mizukoshi E, Bosmann M, et al. Kinetics of CD4+ and CD8+ memory T-cell responses during hepatitis C virus rechallenge of previously recovered chimpanzees. J Virol 2003;77(8):4781–93.

[43] Chiappelli F, Kung M, Lee P, et al. Alcohol modulation of human normal T-cell activation, maturation, and migration. Alcohol Clin Exp Res 1995;19:539–44.

[44] Szabo G. Consequences of alcohol consumption on host defence. Alcohol Alcohol 1999; 34:830–41.

[45] Szabo G, Mandrekar P, Dolganiuc A, et al. Reduced alloreactive T-cell activation after alcohol intake is due to impaired monocyte accessory cell function and correlates with elevated IL-10, IL-13, and decreased IFNgamma levels. Alcohol Clin Exp Res 2001;25(12):1766–72.

[46] Kamal SM, Graham CS, He Q, et al. Kinetics of intrahepatic hepatitis C virus (HCV)-specific CD4+ T cell responses in HCV and *Schistosoma mansoni* coinfection: relation to progression of liver fibrosis. J Infect Dis 2004;189(7):1140–50.

[47] Fowler NL, Torresi J, Jackson DC, et al. Immune responses in hepatitis C virus infection: the role of dendritic cells. Immunol Cell Biol 2003;81(1):63–6.

[48] Bain C, Fatmi A, Zoulim F, et al. Impaired allostimulatory function of dendritic cells in chronic hepatitis C infection. Gastroenterology 2001;120:512–24.

[49] Szabo G, Mandrekar P, Dolganiuc A, et al. Reduced alloreactive T-cell activation after alcohol intake is due to impaired monocyte accessory cell function and correlates with elevated IL-10, IL-13, and decreased IFNgamma levels. Alcohol Clin Exp Res 2001;25(12):1766–72.

[50] Encke J, Wands JR. Ethanol inhibition: the humoral and cellular immune response to hepatitis C virus NS5 protein after genetic immunization. Alcohol Clin Exp Res 2000;24(7):1063–9.

[51] Rowan PJ, Tabasi S, Abdul-Latif M, et al. Psychosocial factors are the most common contraindications for antiviral therapy at initial evaluation in veterans with chronic hepatitis C. J Clin Gastroenterol 2004;38(6):530–4.

[52] Okazaki T, Yoshihara H, Suzuki K, et al. Efficacy of interferon therapy in patients with chronic hepatitis C. Comparison between non-drinkers and drinkers. Scand J Gastroenterol 1994; 29(11):1039–43.

[53] Ohnishi K, Matsuo S, Matsutani K, et al. Interferon therapy for chronic hepatitis C in habitual drinkers: comparison with chronic hepatitis C in infrequent drinkers. Am J Gastroenterol 1996; 91(7):1374–9.

[54] Tabone M, Sidoli L, Laudi C, et al. Alcohol abstinence does not offset the strong negative effect of lifetime alcohol consumption on the outcome of interferon therapy. J Viral Hepat 2002; 9(4):288–2894.

[55] Sherman KE, Rouster SD, Mendenhall C, et al. Hepatitis cRNA quasispecies complexity in patients with alcoholic liver disease. Hepatology 1999;30:265–70.

[56] Lavanchy D. Hepatitis B virus epidemiology, disease burden, treatment, and current and emerging prevention and control measures. J Viral Hepat 2004;11(2):97–107.

[57] Centers for Disease Control and Prevention (CDC). Incidence of acute hepatitis B—United States, 1990–2002. MMWR Morb Mortal Wkly Rep 2004;51–52:1252-4.

[58] Larkin J, Clayton MM, Liu J, et al. Chronic ethanol consumption stimulates hepatitis B virus gene expression and replication in transgenic mice. Hepatology 2001;34(4 Pt 1):792–7.

[59] Nomura H, Hayashi J, Kajiyama W, et al. Alcohol consumption and seroconversion from hepatitis B e antigen in the Okinawa Japanese. Fukuoka Igaku Zasshi 1996;87(11):237–41.

[60] Kondili LA, Tosti ME, Szklo M, et al. The relationships of chronic hepatitis and cirrhosis to alcohol intake, hepatitis B and C, and delta virus infection: a case–control study in Albania. Epidemiol Infect 1998;121(2):391–5.

[61] Corrao G, Torchio P, Zambon A, et al. Exploring the combined action of lifetime alcohol intake and chronic hepatotropic virus infections on the risk of symptomatic liver cirrhosis. Eur J Epidemiol 1998;14(5):447–56.

[62] Murata T, Takanari H, Watanabe S, et al. Enhancement of chronic viral hepatitic changes

by alcohol intake in patients with persistent HBs-antigenemia. Am J Clin Pathol 1990;94(3): 270–3.

[63] Nomura H, Kashiwagi S, Hayashi J, et al. An epidemiologic study of effects of alcohol in the liver in hepatitis B surface antigen carriers. Am J Epidemiol 1988;128(2):277–84.

[64] Montalto G, Cervello M, Giannitrapani L, et al. Epidemiology, risk factors, and natural history of hepatocellular carcinoma. Ann N Y Acad Sci 2002;963:13–20.

[65] Yu MW, Hsu FC, Sheen IS, et al. Prospective study of hepatocellular carcinoma and liver cirrhosis in asymptomatic chronic hepatitis B virus carriers. Am J Epidemiol 1997;145(11): 1039–47.

[66] Hassan MM, Hwang LY, Hatten CJ, et al. Risk factors for hepatocellular carcinoma: synergism of alcohol with viral hepatitis and diabetes mellitus. Hepatology 2002;36(5):1206–13.

[67] Donato F, Gelatti U, Tagger A, et al. Intrahepatic cholangiocarcinoma and hepatitis C and B virus infection, alcohol intake, and hepatolithiasis: a case-control study in Italy. Cancer Causes Control 2001;12(10):959–64.

[68] Tsai JF, Jeng JE, Chuang LY, et al. Habitual betel quid chewing as a risk factor for cirrhosis: a case–control study. Medicine (Baltimore) 2003;82(5):365–72.

[69] Wang LY, You SL, Lu SN, et al. Risk of hepatocellular carcinoma and habits of alcohol drinking, betel quid chewing and cigarette smoking: a cohort of 2416 HBsAg-seropositive and 9421 HBsAg-seronegative male residents in Taiwan. Cancer Causes Control 2003;14(3): 241–50.

[70] Poynard T, Mathurin P, Lai CL, et al. PANFIBROSIS Group. A comparison of fibrosis progression in chronic liver diseases. J Hepatol 2003;38(3):257–65.

[71] Martin-Carbonero L, Benhamou Y, Puoti M, et al. Incidence and predictors of severe liver fibrosis in human immunodeficiency virus-infected patients with chronic hepatitis C: a European collaborative study. Clin Infect Dis 2004;38(1):128–33.

[72] Tural C, Fuster D, Tor J, et al. Time on antiretroviral therapy is a protective factor for liver fibrosis in HIV and hepatitis C virus (HCV) co-infected patients. J Viral Hepat 2003;10(2): 118–25.

[73] Benhamou Y, Di Martino V, Bochet M, et al. Factors affecting liver fibrosis in human immunodeficiency virus-and hepatitis C virus-coinfected patients: impact of protease inhibitor therapy. Hepatology 2001;34(2):283–7.

[74] Bonacini M. Liver injury during highly active antiretroviral therapy: the effect of hepatitis C coinfection. Clin Infect Dis 2004;38(Suppl 2):S104–8.

[75] Martin-Carbonero L, Nunez M, Gonzalez-Lahoz J, et al. Incidence of liver injury after beginning antiretroviral therapy with efavirenz or nevirapine. HIV Clin Trials 2003;4(2):115–20.

[76] Puoti M, Spinetti A, Ghezzi A, et al. Mortality for liver disease in patients with HIV infection: a cohort study. J Acquir Immune Defic Syndr 2000;24(3):211–7.

[77] Rosenthal E, Poiree M, Pradier C, et al. GERMIVIC Joint Study Group. Mortality due to hepatitis C-related liver disease in HIV-infected patients in France (Mortavic 2001 study). AIDS 2003;17(12):1803–9.

[78] Gilbert A, Grenet A. Cirrhose alcoolique hypertrophique pigmentaire. C R Soc Biol 1896;10: 1078–108.

[79] Feder JN, Gnirke A, Thomas W, et al. A novel MHC class I-like gene is mutated in patients with hereditary haemochromatosis. Nat Genet 1996;13:399–408.

[80] Deugnier YM, Turlin B, Powell LW, et al. Differentiation between heterozygotes and homozygotes in genetic hemochromatosis by means of a histological hepatic iron index: a study of 192 cases. Hepatology 1993;17(1):30–4.

[81] Moirand R, Kerdavid F, Loreal O, et al. Regulation of ferritin expression by alcohol in a human hepatoblastoma cell line and in rat hepatocyte cultures. J Hepatol 1995;23(4):431–9.

[82] Suzuki Y, Saito H, Suzuki M, et al. Up-regulation of transferrin receptor expression in hepatocytes by habitual alcohol drinking is implicated in hepatic iron overload in alcoholic liver disease. Alcohol Clin Exp Res 2002;26(8 Suppl):26S–31S.

[83] Valerio Jr LG, Parks T, Petersen DR. Alcohol mediates increases in hepatic and serum nonheme

iron stores in a rat model for alcohol-induced liver injury. Alcohol Clin Exp Res 1996; 20(8):1352–61.

[84] Caro AA, Cederbaum AI. Oxidative stress, toxicology, and pharmacology of CYP2E1. Annu Rev Pharmacol Toxicol 2004;44:27–42.

[85] Wu D, Cederbaum AI. Removal of glutathione produces apoptosis and necrosis in HepG2 cells overexpressing CYP2E1. Alcohol Clin Exp Res 2001;25(4):619–28.

[86] Castillo T, Koop DR, Kamimura S, et al. Role of cytochrome P-450 2E1 in ethanol-, carbon tetrachloride- and iron-dependent microsomal lipid peroxidation. Hepatology 1992;16(4): 992–6.

[87] Nieto N, Friedman SL, Cederbaum AI. Stimulation and proliferation of primary rat hepatic stellate cells by cytochrome P450 2E1-derived reactive oxygen species. Hepatology 2002; 35(1):62–73.

[88] Brittenham GM, Tsukamoto H, Horne W, et al. Experimental liver cirrhosis induced by alcohol and iron. J Clin Invest 1995;96(1):620–30.

[89] Gardi C, Arezzini B, Fortino V, et al. Effect of free iron on collagen synthesis, cell proliferation and MMP-2 expression in rat hepatic stellate cells. Biochem Pharmacol 2002;64(7):1139–45.

[90] Kukielka E, Cederbaum AI. Ferritin stimulation of lipid peroxidation by microsomes after chronic ethanol treatment: role of cytochrome P4502E1. Arch Biochem Biophys 1996;332(1): 121–7.

[91] Tector AJ, Olynyk JK, Britton RS, et al. Hepatic mitochondrial oxidative metabolism and lipid peroxidation in iron-loaded rats fed ethanol. Lab Clin Med 1995;126(6):597–602.

[92] Olynyk J, Hall P, Reed W, et al. A long-term study of the interaction between iron and alcohol in an animal model of iron overload. J Hepatol 1995;22(6):671–6.

[93] Fletcher LM, Dixon JL, Purdie DM, et al. Excess alcohol greatly increases the prevalence of cirrhosis in hereditary hemochromatosis. Gastroenterology 2002;122(2):281–9.

[94] Adams PC, Agnew S. Alcoholism in hereditary hemochromatosis revisited: prevalence and clinical consequences among homozygous siblings. Hepatology 1996;23(4):724–7.

[95] Scotet V, Merour MC, Mercier AY, et al. Hereditary hemochromatosis: effect of excessive alcohol consumption on disease expression in patients homozygous for the C282Y mutation. Am J Epidemiol 2003;158(2):129–34.

[96] Gordeuk VR. African iron overload. Semin Hematol 2002;39(4):263–9.

[97] Gordeuk V, Mukiibi J, Hasstedt S, et al. Iron overload in Africa. Interaction between a gene and dietary iron content. N Engl J Med 1992;326(2):95–100.

[98] Gordeuk VR, Caleffi A, Corradini E, et al. Iron overload in Africans and African-Americans and a common mutation in the SCL40A1 (ferroportin 1) gene. Blood Cells Mol Dis 2003;31(3): 299–304.

[99] Moyo VM, Makunike R, Gangaidzo IT. African iron overload and hepatocellular carcinoma (HA-7-0-080). Eur J Haematol 1998;60(1):28–34.

[100] Moyo VM, Gangaidzo IT, Gordeuk VR, et al. Tuberculosis and iron overload in Africa: a review. Cent Afr J Med 1997;43(11):334–9.

[101] Grundy SM. Metabolic complications of obesity. Endocrine 2000;13(2):155–65.

[102] Haque M, Sanyal AJ. The metabolic abnormalities associated with non-alcoholic fatty liver disease. Best Pract Res Clin Gastroenterol 2002;16(5):709–31.

[103] Ludwig J, Viggiano TR, McGill DB, et al. Nonalcoholic steatohepatitis: Mayo Clinic experiences with a hitherto unnamed disease. Mayo Clin Proc 1980;55(7):434–8.

[104] Falchuk KR, Fiske SC, Haggitt RC, et al. Pericentral hepatic fibrosis and intracellular hyalin in diabetes mellitus. Gastroenterology 1980;78(3):535–41.

[105] Powell EE, Cooksley WG, Hanson R, et al. The natural history of nonalcoholic steatohepatitis: a follow-up study of forty-two patients for up to 21 years. Hepatology 1990;11(1):74–80.

[106] Lindor KD, Kowdley KV, Heathcote EJ, et al. Ursodeoxycholic acid for treatment of nonalcoholic steatohepatitis: results of a randomized trial. Hepatology 2004;39(3):770–8.

[107] Promrat K, Lutchman G, Uwaifo GI, et al. A pilot study of pioglitazone treatment for nonalcoholic steatohepatitis. Hepatology 2004;39(1):188–96.

[108] Flanagan DE, Moore VM, Godsland IF, et al. Alcohol consumption and insulin resistance in young adults. Eur J Clin Invest 2000;30:297–301.

[109] Davies MJ, Baer DJ, Judd JT, et al. Effects of moderate alcohol intake on fasting insulin and glucose concentrations and insulin sensitivity in postmenopausal women: a randomized controlled trial. JAMA 2002;287:2559–62.

[110] Dixon JB, Bhathal PS, O'Brien PE. Nonalcoholic fatty liver disease: predictors of nonalcoholic steatohepatitis and liver fibrosis in the severely obese. Gastroenterology 2001;121(1):91–100.

[111] Laine F, Bendavid C, Moirand R, et al. Prediction of liver fibrosis in patients with features of the metabolic syndrome regardless of alcohol consumption. Hepatology 2004;39(6):1639–46.

[112] Ioannou GN, Weiss NS, Kowdley KV, et al. Is obesity a risk factor for cirrhosis-related death or hospitalization? A population-based cohort study. Gastroenterology 2003;125(4):1053–9.

ELSEVIER
SAUNDERS

CLINICS IN
LIVER DISEASE

Clin Liver Dis 9 (2005) 103–134

Treatment of Alcoholic Hepatitis

Robert S. O'Shea, MD, MSCE[a],*, Arthur J. McCullough, MD[b]

[a]Department of Gastroenterology and Hepatology A30, Cleveland Clinic Foundation,
9500 Euclid Avenue, Cleveland, OH 44195, USA
[b]Division of Gastroenterology, MetroHealth Medical Center, 2500 MetroHealth Drive, Cleveland,
OH 44109; and Case Western Reserve University, Cleveland, OH, USA

Cirrhosis and its sequelae are responsible for close to 2% of all causes of death in the United States [1]. Some studies have suggested that the costs of liver disease may account for as much as 1% of all health care spending [2], with alcohol-related liver disease (ALD) representing a major portion. It accounts for between 40% to 50% of all deaths due to cirrhosis [1], with an accompanying rate of progression of up to 60% in patients with pure alcoholic fatty liver over 10 years [3], and a 5-year survival rate as low as 35% if patients continue to drink [4]. A subset of patients with ALD will develop an acute, virulent form of injury, acute alcoholic hepatitis (AH), which has a substantially worse prognosis. Despite enormous progress in understanding the physiology of this disease, much remains unknown, and therefore, a consensus regarding effective therapy for ALD is lacking. Conventional therapy is still based largely on abstinence from alcohol, as well as general supportive and symptomatic care. Unfortunately, hepatocellular damage may progress despite these measures. Multiple treatment interventions for both the short- and long-term morbidity and mortality of this disease have been proposed, but strong disagreement exists among experts regarding the value of any of the proposed specific therapeutic interventions.

One obstacle to understanding ALD, and the literature describing it, is the heterogeneity of this patient population. As shown in Fig. 1, it has been estimated

Portions of this article appeared previously in McCullough AJ, Fulton S. Treatment of alcoholic hepatitis. Clinics in Liver Disease 1998;2(4):799–819; with permission.

* Corresponding author.
E-mail address: OSHEAR@ccf.org (R.S. O'Shea).

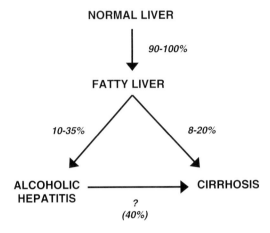

Fig. 1. Outcomes associated with heavy alcohol use.

that although 90% to 100% of heavy drinkers show evidence of fatty liver, only 10% to 35% develop AH, and 8% to 20% develop cirrhosis. Moreover, the severity of illness in these patients is highly variable; the mortality rate in patients hospitalized for AH ranges from 0% to 100% among published trials. The complexity of the disease process—involving immune factors, metabolic components, genetic, and comorbid conditions—has contributed to the failure to fully understand the natural course and pathogenesis of alcohol-induced hepatic injury, which is a major reason for the lack of effective therapies.

Pathogenesis of alcoholic liver disease

AH is a well-characterized histologic disease, defined by a constellation of features, including confluent parenchymal necrosis, varying degrees of steatosis, deposition of intrasinusoidal and pericentral collagen, and infiltration of the liver by polymorphonuclear cells, typically clustered around cytoplasmic structures known as Mallory bodies [5]. Although multiple mechanisms have been proposed, it is clear that the hepatotoxicity of alcohol is mediated by direct and indirect mechanisms, balanced against the liver's ability to regenerate. Because the focus of this review is treatment, pathophysiology is discussed only as it relates to the rationale for specific therapies. In addition to the mechanisms of injury, any number of which may be occurring simultaneously, there are also predisposing factors. Because only 8% to 20% of alcoholics develop cirrhosis and no more than 30% of baboons chronically fed alcohol develop cirrhosis, there must be risk factors that influence individual susceptibility to alcohol's hepatotoxic effects [6–10].

Some of the more established risk factors and their mechanisms are listed in Table 1.

Table 1
Alcoholic liver disease

	Pathogenetic mechanisms	
Risk factors	Direct	Indirect
Gender	Membrane damage	Endotoxin/cytokine
Hepatitis C	Oxidative stress	Immunologic mechanisms
Genetic	Hypermetabolic state	Fibrogenesis
Obesity		
High fat (PUFA) diet		
Malnutrition		
	Impaired hepatic regeneration	

Abbreviation: PUFA, polyunsaturated fatty acid.

One of the most important of these risk factors relevant to the treatment of ALD is the presence of concomitant infection with hepatitis C virus (HCV). Unlike hepatitis B, HCV appears to play an important pathophysiologic role in some patients with ALD [11–13]. Although the results vary somewhat by geography and time, there is a high prevalence of antibodies to HCV among patients with ALD, and the prevalence of HCV infection correlates with the histologic severity of liver disease [14]. There is consistent evidence from natural history studies that the rate of fibrosis progression in patients with chronic hepatitis C correlates strongly with the amount of alcohol ingestion as well [15,16]. Fig. 2 shows the relationship observed in one cross-sectional study that investigated histologic features in patients with chronic hepatitis C; other in-

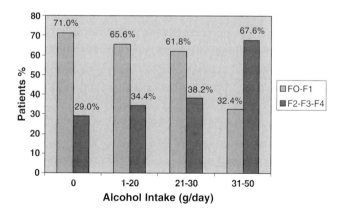

Fig. 2. Likelihood of advanced fibrosis in patients with chronic hepatitis C, based on alcohol intake: corticosteroids used for 1 month decrease the short-term mortality in patients with severe alcoholic liver disease (*$P < 0.01$), as shown in the two most recent prospective studies [16,95]. (*Data from* a cross-sectional study in 260 hepatitis C patients undergoing liver biopsy, questioned regarding lifetime alcohol intake. Fibrosis scored according to Metavir system. *From* Hezode C, Lonjon I, Roudot-Thorval F, et al. Impact of moderate alcohol consumption on histological activity and fibrosis in patients with chronic hepatitis C, and specific influence of steatosis. Aliment Pharmacol Ther 2003;17:1031–7.)

vestigators, using data pooled from large cohort studies, have derived rates of progression of fibrosis based on alcohol intake [15,16].

Furthermore, alcoholic patients with HCV infection have decreased survival rates when compared with alcoholic patients who are not infected. Although HCV infection appears to be an important factor contributing to the severity of ALD, HCV is present in the minority of noncirrhotic ALD patients, and HCV viremia (presence of HCV RNA) should be confirmed if antibodies to HCV are present [17]. It may also be necessary to perform a liver biopsy to separate HCV-induced liver disease in an alcoholic from alcohol-induced liver disease in a patient with superimposed HCV. Consequently, patients with ALD should be screened for HCV and consideration be given to antiviral therapy, especially in those who have histology consistent with chronic viral hepatitis. The likelihood of developing a sustained virologic response, however, is partially based on becoming abstinent from alcohol use.

Therapy for alcoholic hepatitis

Alcoholic liver disease may be considered in terms of both short- and long-term aspects. The therapies for each of these are different, as the pathology and pathophysiology of the two, although intertwined, are different enough to require separate consideration. The focus of this review is on acute AH; long-term management of ALD is addressed elsewhere.

Prognosis

The mortality rate of hospitalized patients with AH varies widely. Based on clinical experience, it is clear that patients with mild disease need not be treated with extraordinary measures. It also is likely that patients with severe disease *in extremis* may be too ill to respond to any form of medical therapy. Consequently, it is important to identify those patients who might benefit from aggressive intervention, as well as those for whom the therapeutic benefit to risk ratio is unfavorable. In addition to allowing the clinician to tailor therapy according to disease severity in an individual patient, predictors of severity may allow a more accurate evaluation of new therapies in patients with disease of similar severity.

Hepatic inflammation

Histologic findings have been shown to add discriminatory ability in patients with AH in several studies. The presence of hepatic inflammation, necrosis, and Mallory bodies appears to be the single most important prognostic histologic factor [18–20], and helps to differentiate patients at high risk of death from others without inflammatory changes [21]. In a study of 217 patients (140 cirrhotics and 77 noncirrhotics) with biopsy-proven ALD [21], the presence of hepatitis indicated a poor prognosis. Patients with cirrhosis and hepatitis had increased

1- and 5-year mortality rates of 27% and 47%, in contrast with cirrhotic patients without hepatitis, who had a survival rate similar to patients with no cirrhosis or hepatitis. These data have been indirectly confirmed by a recent study [22] that found the presence of polymorphonuclear cells on liver biopsy to be a prognostic factor for early and late survival. The extent of infiltration with polymorphonuclear cells has also been shown to correlate with survival in patients treated with steroids [22]. The degree of tissue cholestasis has also been shown to be prognostically important, with increasingly severe cholestasis a marker for poorer prognosis [23].

This relationship is emphasized by the association between hepatic inflammation and continued alcohol use. In a small series from Atlanta [24], serial biopsies were performed in 61 patients with AH but without fibrosis on liver biopsy. If alcohol use continued, 38% of patients progressed to cirrhosis, with AH persisting in the remainder. No patient normalized his or her histology. Abstinence from alcohol did not guarantee complete recovery. Only 27% of abstaining patients had histologic normalization and 18% progressed to cirrhosis. The remaining abstainers had persistent AH when followed for up to 14 months. These findings indicate that the histologic lesion of AH resolves slowly and in a fashion that is related to, but not totally dependent on, continued alcoholic consumption.

Although several clinical scoring systems have been derived in patients with cirrhosis, relatively few have been specifically tested in AH. These indices have used a variety of factors (see Tables 2–4) to predict outcome, with varying success. They have included markers of hepatic metabolic activity, routinely collected biochemical parameters, clinical, and demographic features, or derived scores based on hepatic histology. These severity of illness scores for ALD include the Child-Turcotte-Pugh score, which is used commonly to stage the severity of cirrhosis [25], the combined clinical laboratory index of the University

Table 2
Child-Turcotte classification (Pugh's modification)[a]

	Points		
	1	2	3
Encephalopathy	0	1–2	3–4
Ascites	None	Slight	Moderate
Bilirubin (mg/dL)	1–2	2–3	>3
Albumin (g/dL)	Œ3.5	2.8–3.5	<2.8
Prothrombin time (see prolonged)	1–4	4–6	>6
	Grade	Total score points	
	A	5–6	
	B	7–9	
	C	10–15	

[a] Original classification used malnutrition in place of prothrombin time.

Table 3
Combined clinical and laboratory index (CCLI)[a]

Clinical abnormalities			Laboratory abnormalities		
	Grade	Score		Grade	Score
Encephalopathy	1–3	2	Prothrombin time (sec. over control)	4–5	1
				> 5	2
Collateral	1–2	1	Hemoglobin (% of normal)	75–89.9	1
Circulation	3	3		< 75	3
Edema	1	1	Albumin (g/dL)	2.5–2.9	2
	2–3	2		< 2.5	3
Ascites	1–3	2	Bilirubin (g/dL)	2.1–8	2
				> 8	3
Spider nevi	> 10	1	Alkaline phosphatase (U/dL)	> 330	2
Weakness	—	1			
Anorexia	—	1			

[a] The CCLI score ranges between 0 and 25.

of Toronto [26], the Maddrey discriminant function or the Maddrey Index [27], the Beclere model [22], and, most recently, the MELD score [28].

The Maddrey score was derived in clinical trials of patients with AH, and has since been widely applied clinically in managing patients with AH. It has been used to stratify patients' severity of illness for most of the research involving the use of steroids in patients with AH. In combination with the presence of encephalopathy, a "Discriminant function score" of > 32 is highly correlated with a > 50% short-term mortality rate in patients with AH. Although it is a continuous measure, its interpretation (using a threshold of < or > 32) has converted it into an essentially categorical method of classification. It thus suffers from a related measurement problem, that is, that once patients have exceeded that threshold, they cannot be further characterized without the use of an alternative clinical prediction rule.

Many other studies have attempted to derive more sensitive predictors, testing multiple markers that may play a role in the pathophysiology of the disease. These include clinical features (presence of encephalopathy [26] or new onset ascites [29] or renal failure [30]) demographics (age [31], female gender [32], years of drinking [33]), laboratory studies (hemoglobin level [26], vitamin B12 levels [34], alkaline phosphatase [33], arterial ketone body ratio [35], prothrombin time [26], creatinine [22], bilirubin, or change in bilirubin [36], or factor

Table 4
Maddrey criteria

Discriminant function	Score indicating poor prognosis
Initial	
[4.63 prothrombin time (seconds)] + serum bilirubin (mg/dL)	> 93
Modified	
4.6 (patient's prothrombin time — control time) + serum bilirubin (mg/dL)	> 32

V levels [37]), histologic features on liver biopsy (polymorphonuclear count [22], extent of steatosis [33] or cholestasis [23], presence of megamitochondria [38]), and markers of inflammation and cytokine activity (tumor necrosis factor alpha [TNF-α] levels [39], levels of interleukin [IL]6, 8, 10 [40], lipopolysaccharide binding protein [40], C reactive protein [41], presence of DIC [41], or serum endotoxin levels [40]).

A great deal of work has focused on markers for the abnormal cytokine milieu in these patients. TNF-α levels have not been shown consistently to predict the outcome of this disease, but levels of soluble TNF receptor has been shown to correlate with a linearly increased risk of mortality [42]. Other investigators have examined the role of other cytokines or markers of fibrosis, including serum laminin and type IV collagen [43], as well as YKL-40 and PIIINP (although the contribution of these in patients with pure AH was less clear than in patients with AH superimposed on significant fibrosis/cirrhosis [44]. IL6 concentrations have been shown to correlate with the severity of illness, as measured by the Maddrey discriminant formula, and decrease as patients improved clinically over time (along with levels possibly mediated by IL6, including C-reactive protein) [45]. Soluble intercellular adhesion molecule-1, which mediates the migration of leukocytes, has been shown to correlate with histologic severity of AH [46]. The presence of a leukemoid reaction has been suggested to convey a worse prognosis [47], as has the finding of an elevated arterial blood ketone body ratio (of acetoacetate to 3-hydroxy butyrate) within 48 hours of hospital admission [35]. The hepaplastin time has been shown to correlate with prognosis as part of two risk indices derived in Japan [41,48].

Markers of inflammation related to reactive oxygen intermediates as prognostic indices were tested in a study of whole blood chemiluminescence in patients with AH, and found to correlate closely with the usual indices above, as well as with clinical outcome [49].

More recently, investigators have applied the MELD score to predict the outcome in patients with AH. The MELD score was initially developed to predict outcome in patients undergoing transjugular intrahepatic portal-systemic shunt (TIPS) procedure, and later shown to predict outcome in patients waiting for liver transplant [28]. In a comparison to the use of the discriminant function in patients with AH, the MELD score was shown to predict the outcome as well as the discriminant function (DF) [29]. Using the usual cut points (eg, discriminant function score of > or < 32, versus a MELD score of >11), the two indices had similar sensitivities, although the MELD score may have had a higher specificity.

Dynamic models, which incorporate the changes in laboratory studies over time, have also been used to estimate the outcome in this patient group. Recently, a French group identified the change in bilirubin in the first week of hospitalization to be significantly associated with outcome of patients with AH treated with prednisolone [36].

Although many investigators have studied prognostic features, or derived predictive indices, relatively few of these indices have been independently validated. One review compared the CPT score and the Orrego score with the

Table 5
Clinical trials of steroids in patients with alcoholic hepatitis

Author	Date	Number of patients	Deaths: placebo (with 95% CI)	Deaths: steroid (with 95% CI)	RR
Porter	1971	20	7/9 (0.77) (0.44–0.93)	6/11 (0.55) (0.28–0.79)	1
Helman	1971	37	6/17(0.35) (0.14–0.62)	1/20 (0.05) (0.0013–0.25)	0.143
Campra	1973	45	9/25(0.36) (0.2–0.56)	7/29 (0.35) (0.18–0.57)	1
Blitzer	1977	33	5/16 (0.31) (0.14–0.56)	6/12 (0.5) (0.25–0.75)	1
Lesesne	1978	14	7/7 (1.0) (0.63–1.0)	2/7 (0.29) (0.09–0.65)	0.29
Shumaker	1978	27	7/15 (0.47) (0.25–0.70)	6/12 (0.5) (0.25–0.75)	1
Maddrey	1978	55	6/31 (0.194) (0.09–0.36)	1/24 (0.042) (0.009–0.20)	0.22
Depew	1980	28	7/13 (0.54) (0.29–0.77)	8/15 (0.53) (0.3–0.75)	1
Theodossi	1982	55	16/28 (0.57) (0.39–0.74)	17/27(0.63) (0.44–0.79)	1
Mendenhall	1984	178	50/88 (0.57) (0.46–0.67)	55/90 (0.61) (0.51–0.71)	1
Bories	1987	45	2/21 (0.095) (0.029–0.29)	1/24 (0.042) (0.0098–0.20)	1
Carithers	1989	66	11/31 (0.36) (0.21–0.53)	2/35 (0.057) (0.018–0.19)	0.16
Ramond	1992	61	16/29 (0.55) (0.37–0.72)	4/32 (0.125) (0.05–0.28)	0.23

discriminant function of prothrombin time and bilirubin (see Table 5) in a Veterans Administration Cooperative AH Study, evaluating their ability to predict 30-day mortality [50]. All three correlated with survival, but the less complex Maddrey criteria had the best correlation and highest positive predictive value. Furthermore, the prognostic value of the modified Maddrey criteria has been confirmed prospectively.

The discriminatory ability of the Maddrey score was tested specifically against a model derived from a neural network using nine variables, including five laboratory features, and four clinical variables: albumin, white count, creatinine, bilirubin, prothrombin time, along with the presence of encephalopathy, gastrointestinal bleeding, peritonitis, and ascites. Receiver operator characteristics (ROC) curve areas suggested that the neural network model was significantly more sensitive; adding parameters from day 7 in the hospital suggested even greater ability to determine outcomes. This model, however, has not been widely applied, due in part to its mathematical and practical complexity [51]. As a result, the Maddrey discriminant formula is still widely used by physicians to predict the outcome of patients with acute AH.

Therapeutic agents

Many therapeutic agents have been tested for the treatment of acute AH. Although no review in this area can be exhaustive, the various interventions that have been commonly used are discussed individually below. Our goal is to present an historic overview based on current understanding of the pathophysiology of this disease, as well as to understand the rationale for the current generation of treatments. All authorities agree that abstinence from alcohol is the cornerstone in the long-term management of these patients [32,52–55], with a great deal of evidence to show improvement in outcome in those who become abstinent versus those who continue to drink. Consequently, abstinence should be emphasized, and early diagnosis sought to optimize the beneficial effect of abstinence. Specific interventions for acute AH are discussed below.

Corticosteroids

Rationale

Since the initial publication of histologic studies of patients with this disease, it has been clear that inflammation plays an important role in the outcome. Attempts to treat AH, therefore, have centered on interventions that might address some of the many abnormalities in both humoral and cell-mediated immunity in patients with AH. The specific rationale for the use of corticosteroids is to suppress an overly aggressive immune system provoked by enhanced generation of neo-antigens, including liver-specific lipoprotein, liver membrane antigen, Mallory bodies, and epitopes of protein–aldehyde adducts in the liver [56–58]. Specific immune targets that have been implicated include malondialdehyde and acetaldehyde protein adducts [59]. autoantibodies to P4502E1 and P4503A4 [60], and antibodies to liver membrane antigen [61]. Steroids also exert a direct antifibrotic effect by suppressing the expression of extracellular matrix proteins in the liver.

Corticosteroids also have established anti-inflammatory effects that may directly impact the pathophysiology of this disease. The role of gut derived endotoxin in the stimulation of cytokine (IL1, 6, 8, and TNF)-mediated hepatic damage recently has been emphasized in the pathophysiology of ALD [62–65]. Because cytokine synthesis has been shown to be a highly regulated event with an inhibitory feedback loop provided by glucocorticoids, the effect of steroids in AH, in part, may be related to their inhibition of cytokine production [66].

Clinical trials

Corticosteroids have been used in the treatment of this disorder for several decades, and are thus the most extensively studied treatment modality. Their efficacy, however, remains controversial. Five randomized clinical trials suggested that corticosteroids reduce mortality compared with placebo, whereas eight others found no difference in outcome [67–79].

Although the results are inconsistent, multiple differences in trial design may explain the differing outcomes. These include differences in dose and duration of therapy, selection of patients (eg, varying time intervals before randomization, or inconsistent use of disease severity scoring), possible misclassification bias (eg, differing percentages of patients who underwent liver biopsy to confirm the diagnosis), severity of illness, concomitant medical problems, or medications, as well as undiagnosed chronic viral hepatitis infections, and so on. Despite these differences, three separate meta-analyses have found a benefit to the use of steroids [80–82], and one has suggested no improvement, after attempting to control for potential confounders [83].

The results of the combined data from one of these meta-analyses [82] indicate that corticosteroids should perhaps be targeted to specific subsets of patients

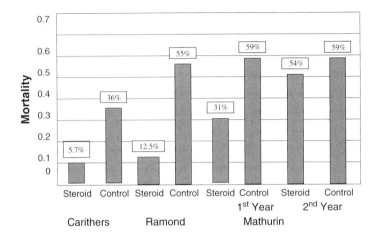

Fig. 3. Corticosteroids used for 1 month also decrease mortality (*$P < 0.01$) at 1 year, but not 2 years, following the discontinuation of corticosteroids. (*Data from* Mathurin P, Duchattelle V, Raymond JM, et al. Survival and prognostic factors in patients with severe alcoholic hepatitis treated with prednisone. Gastroenterology 1996;110:1847–53.)

with severe disease. For example, in one meta-analysis, steroid treatment provided a protective efficacy of 27% in subjects with hepatic encephalopathy, which increased to 44% among higher quality trials and to 51% in patients without active gastrointestinal bleeding. Among subjects without hepatic encephalopathy, corticosteroids had no protective efficacy, and this lack of efficacy was consistent across all trial groups. Fig. 3 presents the results of three trials of steroids used in both the short term (1 month mortality [78,79]) and long term [22]. The impact of steroids on mortality seems consistently greatest in the short term, with no substantial improvement in mortality rates after the first year.

In response to the meta-analysis suggesting a lack of efficacy [83], a reanalysis of pooled data from three placebo-controlled randomized trials, using a uniform measure of disease severity (a Maddrey discriminant formula score > 32) concluded that treated patients had a significantly higher survival than patients given placebo: 84.6% versus 65% [84]. Extrapolating from this result, a number needed to treat of 5 (ie, five patients treated to prevent one death) was calculated. Despite this evidence, physicians remain reluctant to consider steroid treatment, even in the context of severe liver injury [85], and multiple trials have been done without steroids as a comparison treatment.

Practical considerations

These data provide a number of tangible suggestions to the clinician. First, only patients with severe disease (as defined by the presence of hepatic encephalopathy or Maddrey's discriminant function > 32) should be treated with corticosteroids. Second, although such treatment reduces the mortality risk by 25%, there is still a 45% mortality in patients receiving corticosteroids. Consequently, other therapies or combinations therapies need to be investigated. Third, approximately five patients need to be treated to avoid one death. This emphasizes the importance of careful patient selection to avoid the side effects of corticosteroids in the patients who will derive no clinical benefit from them. In general, this means excluding patients with active infection or other strong contraindications to treatment, and being certain of the diagnosis (via liver biopsy if necessary). Histologically confirmed AH correlates poorly with the clinical suspicion of AH [86,87]; up to 28% of patients with a clinical picture of AH do not have histologic features of AH on liver biopsy. Fourth, based on phar-macologic considerations, prednisolone (40 mg/d for 4 weeks then tapered over 2–4 weeks) should be used in favor of prednisone [88].

Supplemental amino acids

Rationale
Protein caloric malnutrition (PCM) is a common finding in alcoholics, in whom ethanol may make up as much as 50% of their caloric intake [89]. It is controversial, however, as to whether poor nutrition is a marker for severity of illness, or a cause in patients with AH. In one study of cirrhotics, nutritional parameters were not found to independently predict mortality [90].

In the largest and most definitive single trial to date, a Veterans Administration Cooperative Study found 100% prevalence of PCM in patients with AH, the severity of which correlated with the degree of liver dysfunction (as measured by bilirubin and prothrombin time) [91]. Furthermore, a composite analysis of PCM correlated with short- and long-term mortality, clinical severity of liver disease, and biochemical hepatic dysfunction. Improved nutritional status also correlated with greater food intake and improved survival. The goal of aggressive nutritional therapy is to supply optimal nutritional replacement to correct pre-existing PCM, while providing sufficient amino acids to encourage hepatic regeneration and normalization without precipitating encephalopathy [92].

Clinical trials
There have been multiple controlled trials published on the use of aggressive nutritional support, including use of standard intravenous amino acid formula-tions as primary therapy for AH. The results of much of the early work are conflicting. As reviewed in [93], several of these studies (see [94–110]) showed improvement in markers of liver function or nutritional parameters, but dif-ferences in clinical outcome have been less impressive (Table 6). Two studies did show an improvement in survival, [98,100], but the remainder concluded that supplemental amino acids offered no survival benefit. As in much of this lit-erature, one caveat is that these studies may have included a large proportion of patients with alcoholic cirrhosis rather than AH, which likely operate via different mechanisms. Moreover, the distinction between effectiveness and efficacy has been commented on in this literature; although patients may have been ran-domized to an intervention, they may not have achieved the outcome. Thus, it is

Table 6
Nutritional support strategies in patients with alcoholic hepatitis

Study	Year	Number of patients	Intervention	Outcome
Lessene	1978	7 study, 7 control	Steroids versus glucose	Seven deaths in glucose group, two in prednisolone group
Galambos	1979	14 patients (non-randomized)	Daily IV enteral hyperalimentation	Improvement in nutritional parameters
Nasrallah	1980	18 control; 17 study	70–85 g IV aminoacids daily × 28 days	Four deaths in control arm, 0 in study arm
Diehl	1985	10 placebo, 5 study	2 L glucose/amino acid solution daily × 30 d	Improvement in nitrogen balance, rate of clinical index improvement, histology
Mendenhall	1985	34 controls, 23 study	Diet high in calories, protein, branched chain amino acids × 30 days	Trend toward decreased mortality in supplemented patients
Calvey	1985	32 controls, 32 intervention	Diet high in calories versus standard diet	No difference in any parameters or clinical outcomes
Naveau	1986	29 study patients, 20 controls	Supplemental 40 kcal/kg/d given IV × 28 days	Greater decrease in total bilirubin in study pts
Soberon	1987	8	Elemental formula diet × 3 days	Improved nitrogen balance, but no difference in survival
Achord	1987	14 control, 14 study	2 L/d IV amino acid and glucose supplement × 21 days	Improvement in histology; no effect on survival or other lfts

Simon	1988	18 control, 16 experimental	PPN × 28 days versus standard diet	No difference in mortality; improved liver tests in PPN group
Cabre	1990	16 study, 19 control diet	Enteral tube feeding × 23 days	47% death rate in controls versus 12% in nutrition group
Bonkovsky	1991	9 / 8 / 10 / 12	PPN × 21 d versus oxandrolone versus Combination versus standard	Improved Child Pugh score
Mezey	1991	28 study, 26 dextrose	2l/d IV amino acid + glucose versus control × 30 days	Improved PT, AST, nitrogen balance but no difference in survival
Kearns	1992	16 patients study, 15 controls	Enteral nutrition supplements (1.5 g/kg protein and 167 kj/kg) × 28 days	No difference in survival, but decreased bili, encephalopathy, improved nitrogen balance in study patients
Mendenhall	1993	137 study, 136 placebo	Oxandrolone + high calorie/protein (60 g protein, 1600 kcal/d) × 30 days versus standard care	No difference in survival overall, but improved in moderately malnourished 19% mortality in study patients versus 51% control
Cabre	2000	35 enteral tube feedings versus 36 steroids	40 mg prednisolone/d versus 2000 kcal/d enteral diet × 28 days	No difference in overall mortality but time of deaths different

difficult to conclude that supplementation is ineffective if nutritional supplementation was not achieved in the treatment group. As an example, in one study the mortality rate was 3.3% in the 30 patients in whom positive nitrogen balance was achieved, but 58% in patients who remained in negative nitrogen balance [110]. These data have not ruled out some benefit to an aggressive nutritinonal approach, and emphasize the need to achieve positive nitrogen balance in such patients.

The most recent study of nutritional intervention compared the use of aggressive nutritional support to the use of steroids, and showed no difference in in-hospital (first month) or overall survival [109], but a decreased mortality rate among patients treated with nutritional therapy who survived the initial hospitalization (8% versus 37%). Most of the deaths in the steroid group were related to infections (9 of 10 in the steroid arm versus 1 of 2 deaths in the nutrition arm). The difference in early versus late mortality rates may be related to different sites of effect of these two interventions. Although technically a negative trial, the similar overall mortality rate suggests a role for nutritional intervention [111].

Practical considerations

Although these trials may not support nutritional therapy as the sole intervention in this disease, there is no evidence to suggest an adverse impact on outcome, or the development of complications such as encephalopathy or ascites. Thus, there is no reason to routinely restrict protein in these patients even if encephalopathy is present. If encephalopathy should worsen with protein feeding, the use of specialized formulation of branched-chain amino acids seems indicated. Specific recommendations for nutritional management have been previously published [112–114].

Promoters of hepatic regeneration

Rationale

The importance of hormonal control of hepatic regeneration has been extensively studied in vitro and in animal experiments. The impetus for these studies has been driven by the hypothesis that alcohol itself, and the inflammation associated with AH may inhibit the regenerative process in damaged hepatocytes [115,116], and hepatocyte proliferation is an important indicator of outcome in AH [117]. There are a number of hormones with clinical potential in this area (including transforming growth factor α, hepatocyte growth factor, epidermal growth factor, glucocorticoids, and growth hormone, as well as thyroid and parathyroid hormones). Insulin and glucagon were the first agents proposed to have regenerative potential, and have been studied extensively, along with several other endogenous hepatotropic substances such as epidermal growth factor (modulated by growth hormone), prostaglandins, and exogenous substances such as malotilate. It also is important to recognize that a suppressed regenerative response of the liver in ALD may be attributed to alterations at the receptor levels for each of these specific hormones. A major limiting factor for the use of growth factors may be decreased binding or downstream events related to specific transcription factors, or the differentiation of progenitor cells [118–120].

Clinical trials

Although the combination of insulin and glucagon has been tried in several clinical situations, the results of five trials have been published using this combination in patients with AH [121–125]. Two of the published trials reported a significant difference or trend for improving survival in favor of I/G therapy [123,124], whereas the others showed no benefit. The treatment has also led to complications—including two deaths in the treated patients related to hypoglycemia. Although a formal meta-analysis has not been done, these data provide no definite evidence that I/G provides a survival advantage in AH.

Given the lack of evidence of efficacy, as well as the potential for significant toxicity, further study regarding improved patient monitoring or other safer hepatotropic substances (such as epidermal growth factor) need to be considered. Epidermal growth factor has been used in experimental models of other liver injury [117–127], but not previously tested in AH.

In addition, several studies of hepatocyte growth factor have been performed in animal models, and showed improvement in outcomes of fatty liver [128] as well as protection from other forms of injury [129]. Given the close association of outcome with the ability of the liver to regenerate, the correlation of hepatocyte growth factor levels with proliferation may promise a therapeutic avenue in this disease [130,131].

The only other regenerative agent used in a clinical trial has been malotilate, which had previously been shown in animal experiments to be protective against ethanol-inhibited hepatocyte regeneration [132]. It also inhibits collagen synthesis by fibroblasts, and inhibits fibroblast migration. Based on these facts, a multicenter European trial was undertaken, which showed a trend toward improved survival in patients treated with one of two doses of malotilate [33], although there was no obvious dose–effect response.

Propylthiouracil

Rationale

The premise for initially using propylthiouracil (PTU) in AH is based on a number of related observations:

1. Acute and chronic alcohol consumption cause a hypermetabolic state characterized by increased energy expenditure and hepatic oxygen consumption in both humans and animals [133–138].
2. Alcohol-related hepatic injury is most evident and severe in the area of the hepatic acinus with the lowest oxygen tension (perivenular Rappaport Zone 3). Alcohol-related injury, therefore, may simulate ischemia related to a relative hypoxia.

3. The use of PTU or surgically induced thyroidectomy partially protects against hypoxic-induced liver injury in animals given ethanol.
4. The severity of liver injury in patients with AH has been correlated with thyroid hormone levels, as has a change in T_3 levels with the likelihood of spontaneous improvement [139].

The fact that hepatic oxygen consumption remains elevated for a relatively short time after alcohol withdrawal (possibly related to adrenergic activity) may have therapeutic implications, suggesting that PTU treatment may have a narrow therapeutic window (10–14 days) following hospitalization and presumed abstinence from alcohol.

Clinical trials

There have been several trials of PTU in patients with ALD, but only two randomized, controlled, double-blind studies investigating short-term PTU therapy in AH.

In a study from the University of Toronto [140], PTU (75 mg every 6 hours for up to 6 weeks) in 19 patients produced a more rapid rate of normalization of the composite Clinical and Laboratory Index (given in Table 3) in patients with biopsy-proven AH. No difference in mortality was observed between the placebo and PTU groups. PTU treatment had no observed effect on patients with fatty liver or with cirrhosis without inflammation.

In the other double-blind controlled trial, from the University of Southern California in 67 patients with severe AH [141], PTU had no significant effect on mortality or laboratory improvement.

A Cochrane systematic review examined the role of PTU in the treatment of alcoholic liver disease, combining the results of these two studies along with others in patients with alcoholic cirrhosis, and concluded that there is no evidence to support the use of PTU in alcoholic liver disease outside of clinical trials [142].

Anabolic steroids

Rationale

Anabolic steroids have been used in alcoholic liver disease for >50 years [143]. The motivation to test these agents came from observational studies of men with ALD, who developed obvious feminization, and later, with specific hormonal testing, were shown to have multiple endocrine abnormalities. In addition, use of these drugs was shown to improve nutritional status in other settings, and in patients with alcoholic fatty liver, to accelerate the disappearance of hepatic steatosis and promote the synthesis of coagulation factors [144]. Significant improvements in catabolic states have been documented, with increases in muscle mass, bone growth, and red cell mass, among others [145,146]. Furthermore, in animal studies, pretreatment with these agents diminished or prevented chemical liver injury, as well as accelerated liver regeneration with improved survival after partial hepatectomy [147]. Consequently, these agents were tested in several trials in ALD, both individually and in combination with other interventions, such as nutritional support, to stimulate hepatic regeneration, protein synthesis, and cell repair, while improving nitrogen retention and energy substrate use [148].

Clinical trials

Five randomized clinical trials [149–154] have tested the benefit of oxandrolone or testosterone in patients with both AH and cirrhosis. In the largest of these, a multicenter, randomized, placebo-controlled VA study, 132 patients with moderate disease and 131 with severe disease were treated with either placebo, prednisolone or oxandrolone (80 mg/d) for 30 days [151]. Although there were no observed differences in the 30-day hospital mortality rates between groups, patients with moderate but not severe disease had improved 6-month survival. The overall survival at follow-up of more than 4 years was not significantly different, but there was a suggestion of benefit in patients with moderate disease who survived longer than 30 days. The reason for stably improved long-term survival without apparent benefit in the acute illness was attributed to the need for stimulation of specific genes, including an increase in fetal gene expression, leading to protein synthesis and sustained hepatic regeneration. On a cautionary note, however, anabolic steroids may compete with glucocorticoids for binding to the glucocorticoid receptor, which may have effects on inflammatory responses [154].

Because anabolic steroids increase protein synthesis and use—a major reason why they were hypothesized to be effective in reversing the nutritional deficiencies in patients with AH—energy and amino acid substrate availability may become rate-limiting factors in these patients. Combination treatment with nutritional therapy was tested in a VA population. The results suggested that oxandrolone combined with amino acids improved liver function in patients with AH as well as survival in patients who were also moderately malnourished, supporting the concept that a combination of therapies may be more efficacious than agents used singly [155]. A large multicenter study of testosterone in male patients with cirrhosis (half of whom also had concomitant AH) in Europe, however, was unable to show any survival benefit, or improvement in liver function [152].

The overall benefit of anabolic steroids in this disease was analyzed in a Cochrane systematic review [156]. That meta-analysis was unable to show a significant improvement in outcome with the use of these drugs, however. Although this does not preclude a benefit, the magnitude of the effect of these agents is presumably small.

Colchicine

Rationale

The inflammatory response of AH is a precursor to fibrosis and eventual cirrhosis. Any impact on the fibrotic process, therefore, might translate into an improved outcome in AH patients. Colchicine has several anti-inflammatory properties, including inhibition of migration of white blood cells, along with collagen production, enhancement of hepatic collagenase activity, and interference with collagen's transcellular movement [157]. Furthermore, it mobilizes hepatic ferritin deposits [158] and may inhibit cytokine production, inflammation, and associated fibroblast proliferation. In animal studies, it has been shown to reduce hepatic necrosis after treatment with carbon tetrachloride [159].

Clinical trials and practical considerations

Two studies have been published reporting on the therapeutic efficacy of colchicine in AH [160,161]. Neither showed a therapeutic benefit, although both studies suffered from significant losses to follow-up (more than 50% in one article [161]). A Cochrane systematic review, which also included several unpublished abstracts, was unable to show any significant improvement in outcome in patients with AH or established cirrhosis treated with colchicine [162].

S-Adenosyl-L-methionine

Rationale

S-Adenosyl-L-methionine (SAMe) is a naturally occurring molecule produced in vivo from methionine and adenosine triphosphate by the enzyme SAMe synthetase. It is an important compound in the synthesis of membrane phospholipids, and also serves as a precursor for the production of glutathione, which in turn, is a major physiologic defense mechanism against oxidative stress. Animal studies have shown that glutathione depletion within hepatic mitochondria sensitizes the liver to alcohol-induced injury, and that restoration of SAMe levels may protect the liver from alcohol liver injury [163,164]. SAMe synthetase activity has been reported to be decreased in cirrhosis [165]. Specific mechanisms include effects on the production of TNF, as well as the levels of anti-inflammatory cytokines, such as IL-10 [166]. The importance of SAMe in ALD was the focus of a National Institutes of Health (NIH)-sponsored symposium in 2001 [167]. Subsequent studies have documented decreased levels of SAMe in patients with AH [168].

Clinical trials

A trial in 62 patients with alcoholic cirrhosis treated with SAMe and followed for up to 2 years was not able to detect a difference in overall mortality in treated patients versus controls. The subgroup with Childs A or B cirrhosis receiving supplementation showed a significant improvement in the rate of liver transplant or mortality, however [169]. A Cochrane systematic review failed to show any significant differences in outcome in patients treated with alcoholic liver disease, but admittedly, the number of patients studied with AH is minimal [170]. In response to the pressing need for further trials [171], an NIH funded study is now underway to evaluate the role of SAMe in patients with moderate AH.

Calcium channel blockers

Loss of regulation of hepatic intracellular calcium has been postulated to play a role in cell injury in a number of clinical situations, including ischemia and reactions to chemical injury [172]. Calcium is a major second messenger involved in cell signaling, and has been shown to play a role in activation of Kupffer cells [173]. The complex relationship of calcium metabolism and oxidative stress suggests a possible avenue of treatment, as several calcium channel blockers have been shown to reduce hypoxic liver injury. Based on animal data demonstrating prevention of AH with calcium channel blockade [174], a clinical trial [175] to test this possibility was undertaken in 32 patients with well-documented AH. Unfortunately, there was no difference in clinical outcome in treated patients versus controls. Although no evidence of effect was noted, however, the sample size was too small to conclude that calcium channel blockers may not have a role in long-term treatment for the prevention of inflammation and fibrosis.

Polyunsaturated lecithin

Rationale

Chronic alcohol consumption produces changes in the phospholipid of cell membranes that may be prevented by supplementation of polyunsaturated phospholipid. It also appears a specific lipid—polyunsaturated lecithin (PUL)—may have two protective mechanisms other than stabilizing membranes. First, PUL may prevent the transformation of lipocytes into collagen-producing transitional cells; second, PUL may increase collagenase activity, which offsets increased collagen production [176].

Clinical trials

A PUL-supplemented liquid diet prevented septal fibrosis and cirrhosis in baboons, while decreasing the activation of lipocytes into collagen-producing transitional cells [177,178]. The mechanism for this is thought to be related to a decrease in oxidative stress [179], possibly related to restoration of SAMe levels [180]. Based on these animal data, a large trial of supplementation with polyenylphosphatidylcholine in 789 veterans was undertaken, who were then followed for 2 years [181]. A follow-up liver biopsy in 412 of them unfortunately did not show any significant difference in the stage of fibrosis in patients on active treatment versus placebo.

Complementary/alternative medicines

A number of studies have investigated herbs and nutritional supplements in patients with alcoholic liver disease, including silymarin, the active ingredient in milk thistle [182]. Based on its possible mechanism of action as an antioxidant, several studies have been undertaken in acute and chronic liver disease, including alcoholic liver disease (reviewed in [183,184]). In animal studies, silymarin has been shown to prevent carbon tetrachloride injury in rats, and possibly to slow the rate of progression of alcoholic liver injury in baboons [185]. Human studies, however, have been less convincing. Two studies have been undertaken in patients with AH [186,187]. In the largest study to date, [186], 200 patients with histologically proven ALD (including 48 with AH) were randomized to receive either silymarin or placebo; no effect on survival was noted at 2 years in the subset of patients with AH or in the larger group with cirrhosis. Similar findings were noted in the Trinchet paper [187], which had randomized 116 patients with AH to either placebo or silymarin.

Other antioxidants have also been tried in patients with AH, including vitamin E, based partly on preliminary studies that suggest a role in nonalcoholic steatohepatitis [188]. Unfortunately, in a recently published long-term trial in 25 patients treated with vitamin E for 3 months, no significant clinical differences were seen compared with patients treated with placebo [189].

Case reports

Several authors have reported results of extremely aggressive interventions in patients with AH. A case series from University College of London reported on the outcome of eight patients who were hospitalized with AH and ultimately treated with a molecular adsorbent recirculating system [190]. Seven of the eight had accompanying hepatorenal syndrome. Five patients survived to discharge, and a 4- to 3-month follow-up, which was substantially better than the predicted outcome. A larger study is ongoing to test the utility of these systems in AH. Perhaps operating by similar principles (ie, correction of an abnormal cytokine and inflammatory milieu), a case report from Japan describes the outcome of one patient with severe AH treated with leukocytapharesis after failing to improve substantially on steroids [191].

A case series from the University of Pittsburgh reviewed the course of 9 patients who had undergone liver transplantation for AH, and found that the overall posttransplant survival was relatively similar to that seen in other patients with end-stage liver disease [192]. Other authors have also published cases of patients successfully transplanted with AH [193]. The long-term outcome of patients who were transplanted with histologic evidence of AH in addition to cirrhosis has not shown consistently any real difference when compared with patients with only cirrhosis seen in the explant [194]. In an accompanying editorial, it was pointed out that the severity of illness of patients with AH was at least as high or higher than other patients with end-stage liver disease, and therefore, there was a need to consider offering a potentially life-saving therapy without a mandatory waiting/abstinence time [195]. In an era of ongoing organ shortage, however, the role for these interventions is not yet clear.

Potential new therapies

The growing understanding of the importance of cytokines in the pathophysiology of AH has led to numerous attempts to intervene, particularly in the TNF pathway. These are discussed below.

Pentoxifylline

Several recent studies have focused on the use of pentoxifylline, a phosphodiesterase inhibitor initially used in the treatment of peripheral vascular disease, based on its ability to increase erythrocyte flexibility, reduce blood viscosity, and inhibit platelet aggregation. Phosphodiesterase inhibition, however, has also been shown to have multiple effects on immune markers. In particular, pentoxifylline has been shown to reduce the production of TNF-α, IL-5, IL-10, and IL-2. It also has been shown to decrease the transcription of IL-2 and TNF-α promoters in transiently transfected normal T cells, to inhibit the activation of nuclear factor-κB (NF-κB) and nuclear factor of activated T cells, and stimulate activator protein-1 and cAMP response element-binding proteins [196]. In animal models, it has been shown to reduce portal pressure in cirrhosis [197,198].

Based on these data, a clinical trial using pentoxifylline in 101 patients with severe acute AH was undertaken [199]. Patients were randomized to receive oral pentoxifylline 400 mg three times daily (n = 49) or placebo (n = 52). The mean duration of treatment in the respective groups was 21.5 and 23 days. In-hospital mortality was significantly lower in pentoxifylline recipients, compared with controls (24.5 versus 46.1% of patients), yielding a relative risk of 0.59. Of the patients who died, hepatic failure with hepatorenal syndrome developed in significantly fewer pentoxifylline recipients, compared with controls (6/12 [50%] versus 22 of 24 [91.7%]). Last, new-onset renal impairment developed in significantly fewer pentoxifylline recipients, compared with controls (5 versus 20 patients); further progression to hepatorenal syndrome occurred in 4 and 18 patients in the respective treatment groups, yielding a relative risk of 0.32. The difference in mortality between the two groups suggests a number needed to treat (NNT) of 4.7 (ie, to prevent one death, 4.7 patients should be treated)—almost identical to the number arrived at by Mathurin et al comparing the use of steroids to placebo. The mechanism whereby pentoxifylline decreased the development of hepatorenal syndrome (HRS) is unclear, but could be related to either direct effects on the liver (through any of the above possible mechanisms), or, alternatively, by a direct renal effect.

These data, along with more recent studies of drugs that specifically oppose particular cytokines, have generated interest in this avenue of treatment, given the potential for decreased risks of infection compared with conventional steroid treatment, and more specific antagonism of the inflammatory pathophysiology of this disease. Several trials using infliximab (a monoclonal chimeric anti-TNF antibody) have been published or presented; unfortunately, these trials were preliminary or pilot studies, not powered to detect clinically important differences. In addition, three were uncontrolled, and none of them used steroids as a comparison arm. Although the results of intermediate markers of liver damage improved in several of these studies, the clinical outcomes did not conclusively show an improvement in survival [200–202].

On the basis of these studies, a clinical trial using infliximab (10 mg/kg) in combination with prednisolone (40 mg/d) versus prednisolone alone was begun in France [203]. A total of 36 patients were randomized before the trial was stopped prematurely by the data safety monitoring board, based on a substantially higher death rate in the infliximab group (39% versus 11%). Most of these were related to a very significant increase in the risk of infection in patients on active treatment compared with controls, who had been treated with prednisolone alone [204].

The design of this study has been faulted as employing too much immunosuppression, including too high a dose of infliximab [205], particularly in combination with steroids, which may have impaired both neutrophil and T cell function, as well as T cell survival. Questions have been also been raised regarding the extent to which TNF inhibition is useful in this disease, as TNF has been shown to be important in hepatic regeneration [206] as well as in alcohol-related liver injury, and therefore, how much TNF inhibition may be helpful, or whether TNF inhibition may become counterproductive.

More recently, several small studies have addressed the use of etanercept, a dimeric fusion protein consisting of the extracellular ligand-binding portion of the human tumor necrosis factor receptor linked to the Fc portion of human IgG1. Etanercept has been marketed for a variety of rheumatologic disorders including rheumatoid and psoriatic arthritis, as well as ankylosing spondylitis. The only published report in patients with liver disease treated 13 patients with moderate or severe AH (defined by a discriminant function value greater than 15 or the presence of spontaneous hepatic encephalopathy) for a 2-week duration [207]. The 30-day survival rate of patients receiving etanercept was 92%. Adverse events (including infection, hepatorenal decompensation, and gastrointestinal bleeding), required premature discontinuation of etanercept in 23% of patients. Based on the results of this study, a larger multicenter controlled trial is now underway.

Although these results are intriguing, the lack of a control arm, the inclusion of patients with relatively more moderate liver disease (making interpretation of survival statistics uncertain), and the high drop out rate temper the enthusiasm for use of etanercept. Moreover, in light of the data from the studies of infliximab, the extent to which complete TNF inhibition (via antibody or receptor blockade) is useful, or how best to measure it, is unclear. The outcome of further clinical trials is desperately needed to answer these questions.

Future directions

Although the recognition of the role of cytokines—and in particular, TNF-α—in the pathophysiology of ALD represents a major advance, much remains

---

Box 1. Proposed approach to management of alcoholic liver disease

Risk stratification (Using Maddrey discriminant function > 32, presence of hepatic encephalopathy, MELD score > 11, or other index).

Low risk:
    (decrease in score or total bilirubin in hospital)
    Supportive care
    Abstinence
    Rehabilitation
    Counselling to prevent recidivism
High risk:
    (clinically worsening)
    Nutritional supplements
    Consider prednisolone or pentoxifylline or other specific
      anticytokine therapies

---

unknown. In particular, emerging data suggests a role for apoptosis in this disease [208,209], and therefore, targeted therapy may evolve in that direction [210].

In light of an incomplete understanding of the pathophysiologic mechanisms involved and conflicting data regarding the efficacy of specific interventional therapies for ALD, a conservative approach seem justified. Although it is difficult to endorse an algorithim for management of patients with alcoholic hepaititis, based on the data reviewed, an approach is outlined in Box 1. This includes general supportive and nutritional care, with aggressive nutritional interventions, and the judicious use of corticosteroids in selected patients with severe illness. In addition, abstinence from alcohol and continuous nutritional monitoring seem prudent on a long-term basis.

Several of the following important issues need to be emphasized.

1. The high prevalence of hepatitis C must be considered, regarding its potential influence upon prognosis and therapeutic strategies.
2. Future therapeutic directions should aim at specific pathophysiologic mechanisms of alcoholic hepatocellular damage as well as the regulation of hepatic regeneration in this disease. Furthermore, combination therapy targeting both direct and indirect mechanisms of alcoholic hepatocellular damage as well as regeneration capacity of the injured liver may prove to be necessary after patient individualization and assessment of disease severity and prognosis.

References

[1] Kim WR, Brown RS, Terrault NA, et al. Burden of liver disease in the United States: summary of a workshop. Hepatology 2002;36:227–42.

[2] Sandler RS, Everhart JE, Donowitz M, et al. The burden of selected digestive diseases in the United States. Gastroenterology 2002;122:1500–11.

[3] Teli MR, Day CP, Burt AD, et al. Determinants of progression to cirrhosis or fibrosis in pure alcoholic fatty liver. Lancet 1995;346(8981):987–90.

[4] Powell Jr WJ, Klatskin G. Duration of survival in patients with Laennec's cirrhosis. Influence of alcohol withdrawal, and possible effects of recent changes in general management of the disease. Am J Med 1968;44(3):406–20.

[5] Hall PD. Pathological spectrum of alcoholic liver disease. Alcohol Alcohol Suppl 1994;2: 303–13.

[6] Lindros KO. Alcoholic liver disease: pathobiological aspects. J Hepatol 1995;23(suppl 1):7–15.

[7] Koch OR, Pani G, Borrello S, et al. Oxidative stress and antioxidant defenses in ethanol-induced cell injury. Mol Aspects Med 2004;25(1–2):191–8.

[8] Degoul F, Sutton A, Mansouri A, et al. Homozygosity for alanine in the mitochondrial targeting sequence of superoxide dismutase and risk for severe alcoholic liver disease. Gastroenterology 2001;120:1468–74.

[9] Monzoni A, Masutti F, Saccoccio G, et al. Genetic determinants of ethanol-induced liver damage. Mol Med 2001;7(4):255–62.

[10] Bellentani S, Saccoccio G, Costa G, et al, and the Dionysos Study Group. Drinking habits as cofactors of risk for alcohol induced liver damage. Gut 1997;41:845–50.

[11] Koff RS, Dienstag JL. Extrahepatic manifestations of hepatitis C and the association with alcoholic liver disease. Semin Liver Dis 1995;15:101–9.

[12] Rigamonti C, Mottaran E, Reale E, et al. Moderate alcohol consumption increases oxidative stress in patients with chronic hepatitis C. Hepatology 2003;38:42–9.

[13] Peters MG, Terrault NA. Alcohol use and hepatitis C. Hepatology 2002;36(5 suppl 1):S220–5.

[14] Tanaka T, Yabusako T, Yamashita T, et al. Contribution of hepatitis C virus to the progression of alcoholic liver disease. Alcohol Clin Exp Res 2000;24(4 suppl):112S–6S.

[15] Poynard T, Bedossa P, Opolon P. Natural history of liver fibrosis progression in patients with chronic hepatitis C: the OBSVIRC, METAVIR, CLINVIR, and DOSVIRC groups. Lancet 1997;349:825–32.

[16] Hezode C, Lonjon I, Roudot-Thoraval F, et al. Impact of moderate alcohol consumption on histological activity and fibrosis in patients with chronic hepatitis C, and specific influence of steatosis: a prospective study. Aliment Pharmacol Ther 2003;17:1031–7.

[17] Befrits R, Hedman M, Blomquist L, et al. Chronic hepatitis C in alcoholic patients: prevalence, genotypes, and correlations to liver disease. Scand J Gastroenterol 1995;30:1113–8.

[18] Bouchier IRD, Hislop WS, Prescott RJ. A prospective study of alcoholic liver disease and mortality. J Hepatol 1992;16:290–7.

[19] Chedid A, Mendenhall CL, Gartside P, et al. Prognostic factors in alcoholic liver disease. Am J Gastroenterol 1991;86:210–6.

[20] Diehl AM. Alcoholic liver disease: natural history. Liver Transplant Surg 1997;3:206–11.

[21] Orrego H, Blake JE, Blendis M, et al. Prognosis of alcoholic cirrhosis in the presence and absence of alcoholic hepatitis. Gastroenterology 1987;92:208–14.

[22] Mathurin P, Duchatelle V, Ramond JM, et al. Survival and prognostic factors in patients with severe alcoholic hepatitis treated with prednisolone. Gastroenterology 1996;110:1847–53.

[23] Nissenbaum M, Chedid A, Mendenhall C, et al, for the VA Cooperative Study Group #119. Prognostic signficance of cholestatic alcoholic hepatitis. Dig Dis Sci 1990;35:891–6.

[24] Galambos JT. Natural history of alcoholic hepatitis: III. Histological changes. Gastroenterology 1972;63:1026–35.

[25] Pugh RWH, Murray-Lyon IM, Dawson JL, et al. Transection of the esophagus for bleeding varices. Br J Surg 1983;60:646–9.

[26] Orrego H, Israel Y, Blake JE, et al. Assessment of prognostic factors in alcoholic liver disease: toward a global quantitative expression of severity. Hepatology 1983;3:805–905.

[27] Maddrey WC. Alcoholic hepatitis: clinicopathologic features and therapy. Semin Liver Dis 1988;8:91–102.

[28] Kamath PS, Wiesner RH, Malinchoc M, et al. A model to predict survival in patients with end-stage liver disease. Hepatology 2001;33(2):464–70.

[29] Sheth M, Riggs M, Patel T. Utility of the Mayo End-Stage Liver Disease (MELD) score in assessing prognosis of patients with alcoholic hepatitis. BMC Gastroenterol 2002;2:1–5.

[30] Garcia RJ, Cutrin PC, Rodriguez AJ, et al. Clinical forms and prognostic criteria in alcoholic hepatitis. Med Int 1989;6:291–4.

[31] Kumashiro R, Sata M, Ishii K, et al. Prognostic factors for short-term survival in alcoholic hepatitis in Japan: analysis by logistic regression. Alcohol Clin Exp Res 1996;20:83–6.

[32] Pares A, Caballeria J, Bruguera M. Histological course of alcoholic hepatitis: influence of abstinence, sex and extent of hepatic damage. J Hepatol 1986;2:33–42.

[33] Keiding S, Badsberg JH, Becker U, et al. The prognosis of patients with alcoholic liver disease: an international randomized placebo-controlled trial on the effects of malotilate on survival. J Hepatol 1994;20:454–60.

[34] Baker H, Frank O, DeAngelis B. Plasma vitamin B12 titres as indicators of disease severity and mortality of patients with alcoholic hepatitis. Alcohol Alcohol 1987;22:1–5.

[35] Saibara T, Maeda S, Onishi S, et al. The arterial blood ketone body ratio as a possible marker of multi-organ failure in patients with alcoholic hepatitis. Liver 1994;14:85–9.

[36] Mathurin P, Abdelnour M, Ramond MJ, et al. Early change in bilirubin levels is an important prognostic factor in severe alcoholic hepatitis treated with prednisolone. Hepatology 2003; 38:1363–9.

[37] Pereira LM, Langley PG, Bird GL, et al. Coagulation factors V and VIII in relation to severity and outcome in acute alcoholic hepatitis. Alcohol Alcohol 1992;27:55–61.

[38] Chedid A, Mendenhall CL, Tosch T, et al. Significance of megamitochondria in alcoholic liver disease. Gastroenterology 1986;90:1858–64.

[39] Bird GL, Sheron N, Goka AK, et al. Increased tumor necrosis factor in severe alcoholic hepatitis. Ann Intern Med 1990;112:917–20.

[40] Fujimoto M, Uemura M, Nakatani Y, et al. Plasma endotoxin and serum cytokine levels in patients with alcoholic hepatitis: relation to severity of liver disturbance. Alcohol Clin Exp Res 2000;24:48S–54S.

[41] Fujimoto M, Uemura M, Kojima H, et al. Prognostic factors in severe alcoholic liver injury. Alcohol Clin Exp Res 1999;23:33S–8S.

[42] Spahr L, Giostra E, Frossard JL, et al. Soluble TNF-R1, but not tumor necrosis factor alpha, predicts the 3-month mortality in patients with alcoholic hepatitis. J Hepatol 2004;41: 229–34.

[43] Castera L, Hartmann DJ, Chapel F, et al. Serum laminin and type IV collagen are accurate markers of histologically severe alcoholic hepatitis in patients with cirrhosis. J Hepatol 2000;32: 412–8.

[44] Nojgaard C, Johansen JS, Christensen E, et al. Serum levels of YKL-40 and PIIINP as prognostic markers in patients with alcoholic liver disease. J Hepatol 2003;39:179–86.

[45] Hill DB, Marsano L, Cohen D, et al. Increased plasma interleukin-6 concentrations in alcoholic hepatitis. J Lab Clin Med 1992;119:547–52.

[46] Douds AC, Lim AG, Jazrawi RP, et al. Serum intercellular adhesion molecule-1 in alcoholic liver disease and its relationship with histological disease severity. J Hepatol 1997;26:280–6.

[47] Mitchell RG, Michael M, Sandidge D. High mortality among patients with the leukemoid reaction and alcoholic hepatitis. South Med J 1991;84:281–2.

[48] Kumashiro R, Sata M, Ishii K, et al. Prognostic factors for short-term survival in alcoholic hepatitis in Japan: analysis by logistic regression. Alcohol Clin Exp Res 1996;20:383A–6A.

[49] Lunel F, Descamps-Latscha B, Descamps D, et al. Predictive value of whole blood chemiluminescence in patients with alcoholic hepatitis. Hepatology 1990;12:264–72.

[50] Mendenhall CL. Alcoholic hepatitis. In: Schiff L, Schiff ER, editors. Diseases of the liver. 6th edition. Philadelphia: JB Lippincott Co.; 1987. p. 669–85.

[51] Lapuerta P, Rajan S, Bonacini M. Neural networks as predictors of outcomes in alcoholic patients with severe liver disease. Hepatology 1997;25:302–6.

[52] Borowsky SA, Strome S, Lott E. Continued heavy drinking and survival in alcoholic cirrhotics. Gastroenterology 1981;80:1405–9.

[53] Brunt PW, Kew MC, Scheuer PJ, et al. Studies in alcoholic liver disease in Britain. Gut 1974;15:52–8.

[54] Kawasaki S, Henderson M, Hertzler G, et al. The role of continued drinking in loss of portal perfusion after distal splenorenal shunt. Gastroenterology 1991;100:799–804.

[55] Powell JH, Klatskin G. Duration of survival in Laënnec's cirrhosis. Am J Med 1968;44: 406–20.

[56] Clot P, Parola M, Bellomo G, et al. Plasma membrane hydroxyethyl radical adducts cause antibody-dependent cytotoxicity in rat hepatocytes exposed to alcohol. Gastroenterology 1997; 113:265–76.

[57] Israel Y. Antibodies against ethanol-derived protein adducts: pathogenetic implications. Gastroenterology 1997;113:353–5.

[58] Ma Y, Gaken J, McFarlane BM, et al. Alcohol dehydrogenase: a target of humoral autoimmune response in liver disease. Gastroenterology 1997;112:483–92.

[59] Tuma DJ. Role of malondialdehyde-acetaldehyde adducts in liver injury. Free Radic Biol Med 2002;32:303–8.

[60] Lytton SD, Helander A, Zhang-gouillon Z, et al. Autoantibodies against cytochromes P-450E1 and P4503A in alcoholics. Mol Pharmacol 1999;55:223–33.

[61] Burt AD, Anthony RS, Hislop WS, et al. Liver membrane antibodies in alcoholic liver disease: 1. Prevalence and immunoglobulin class. Gut 1982;23(3):221–5.

[62] Adams DH, Burra P, Hkubscher SG, et al. Endothelial activation and circulating vascular adhesion molecules in alcoholic liver disease. Hepatology 1994;19:588–94.

[63] Mawet E, Chiratori Y, Hikiba Y, et al. Cytokine-induced neutrophil chemoattractant release from hepatocytes is moduled by kupffer cells. Hepatology 1996;23:353–8.

[64] McClain CJ, Hill D, Schmidt J, et al. Cytokines and alcoholic liver disease. Semin Liver Dis 1993;13:170–82.

[65] McCuskey RS, Nishida J, Eguchi H, et al. Role of endotoxin in the hepatic microvascular inflammatory response to ethanol. J Gastroenterol Hepatol 1995;10:518–23.

[66] Papanicolaou DA, Wilder RL, Manolagas SC, et al. The pathophysiologic roles of Interleukin-6 in human disease. Ann Intern Med 1998;128:127–37.

[67] Helman RA, Temko MH, Nye SW, et al. Natural history and evaluation of prednisolone therapy. Ann Intern Med 1971;74:311–21.

[68] Porter HP, Simon FR, Pope CE, et al. Corticosteroid therapy in severe alcoholic hepatitis. N Engl J Med 1971;284:1350–5.

[69] Campra JL, Hamlin EM, Kirshbaum RJ, et al. Prednisone therapy of acute alcoholic hepatitis. Ann Intern Med 1973;79:625–31.

[70] Blitzer BL, Mutchnick MG, Joshi PH, et al. Adrenocorticosteroid therapy in alcoholic hepatitis: a prospective, double-blind randomized study. Am J Dig Dis 1977;22:477–84.

[71] Lesesne HR, Bozymski EM, Fallon HJ. Treatment of alcoholic hepatitis with encephalopathy. Comparison of prednisolone with caloric supplements. Gastroenterology 1978;74:169–73.

[72] Maddrey WC, Boitnott JK, Bedine MS, et al. Corticosteroid therapy of alcoholic hepatitis. Gastroenterology 1978;75:193–9.

[73] Shumaker JB, Resnick RH, Galambos JT, et al. A controlled trial of 6-methylprednisolone in acute alcoholic hepatitis. Am J Gastroenterol 1978;69:443–9.

[74] Depew W, Boyer T, Omata M, et al. Double-blind controlled trial of prednisolone therapy in patients with severe acute alcoholic hepatitis and spontaneous encephalopathy. Gastroenterology 1980;78:524–9.

[75] Theodossi A, Eddleston ALWF, Williams R. Controlled trial of methylprednisolone therapy in severe acute alcoholic hepatitis. Gut 1982;23:75–9.

[76] Mendenhall CL, Anderson S, Garcia-Pont P, et al. Short-term and long- term survival in patients with alcoholic hepatitis treated with oxandrolone and prednisolone. N Engl J Med 1984;311:1464–70.

[77] Bories P, Guedj JY, Mirouze D, et al. Traitement de l'hépatite alcoolique aiguë par la prednisolone. Presse Med 1987;16:769–72.

[78] Carithers Jr RL, Herlong HF, Diehl AM, et al. Methyiprednisolone therapy in patients with severe alcoholic hepatitis: a randomized multicenter trial. Ann Intern Med 1989;110: 685–90.

[79] Ramond MJ, Poynard T, Rueff B, et al. A randomized trial of prednisolone in patients with severe alcoholic hepatitis. N Engl J Med 1992;326:507–12.

[80] Daures JP, Peray P, Bones P, et al. Place de la corticothérapie dans le traitement des hépatites alcooliques aiguës. Résultats dune métaanalyse. Gastroenterol Clin Biol 1991;15:223–8.

[81] Reynolds TB, Benhamou JP, Blake J, et al. Treatment of alcoholic hepatitis. Gastroenterol Int 1989;2:208–16.

[82] Imperiale TF, McCullough AJ. Do corticosteroids reduce mortality from alcoholic hepatitis? Ann Intern Med 1990;113:299–307.

[83] Christensen E, Gludd C. Glucocorticosteroids are ineffective in alcoholic hepatitis: a meta-analysis adjusting for confounding variables. Gut 1995;37:113–8.

[84] Mathurin P, Mendenhall CL, Carithers RL, et al. Corticosteroids improve short term survival in patients with severe alcoholic hepatitis (AH): individual data analysis of the last three randomized placebo controlled double blind trials of corticosteroids in severe AH. J Hepatol 2002;36:480–7.

[85] O'Keefe C, McCormick PA. Severe acute alcoholic hepatitis: an audit of medical treatment. Ir Med J 2002;95:108–11.

[86] Mathurin P, Duchatelle V, Ramond JM, et al. Survival and prognostic factors in patients with severe alcoholic hepatitis treated with prednisolone. Gastroenterology 1996;110:1847–53.

[87] Schichting P, Juhl E, Poulsen H, et al. Alcoholic hepatitis superimposed on cirrhosis, clinical significance of long term prednisone treatment. Scand J Gastroenterol 1976;22:305–12.

[88] Uribe M, Schalm SW, Summerskill WHJ, et al. Oral prednisone for chronic active liver disease: dose response and bioavailability studies. Gut 1978;19:1131–5.

[89] Lieber CS. Medical disorders of alcoholism. N Engl J Med 1995;333:1058–65.

[90] Merli M, Riggio O, Dally L, et al. Does malnutrition affect survival in cirrhosis. Hepatology 1996;23:1041–6.

[91] Mendenhall CL, Anderson S, Weesner RE, et al. Protein calorie malnutrition associated with alcoholic hepatitis. Am J Med 1984;76:211–22.

[92] McCullough AJ, Tavill AS. Disordered energy and protein metabolism in liver disease. Semin Liver Dis 1991;11:265–77.

[93] Nomnpleggi DJ, Bonkovsky HL. Nutritional supplementation in chronic liver disease: an analytical review. Hepatology 1994;19:518–33.

[94] Achord JL. A prospective randomized clinical trial of peripheral amino acid-glucose supplementation in acute alcoholic hepatitis. Am J Gastroenterol 1987;82:871–5.

[95] Bonkovsky HL, Fiellin DA, Smith GS, et al. A randomized, controlled trial of treatment of alcoholic hepatitis with parenteral nutrition and oxandrolone: I. Short-term effects on liver function. Am J Gastroenterol 1991;86:1200–8.

[96] Diehl AM, Boitnott JK, Herlong HF, et al. Effect of parenteral amino acid supplementation in alcoholic hepatitis. Hepatology 1985;5:57–63.

[97] Mendenhall CL, Moritz TE, Roselle GA, et al. A study of oral nutritional support with oxandrolone in malnourished patients with alcoholic hepatitis: results of a Department of Veterans Affairs Cooperative Study. Hepatology 1993;17:564–76.

[98] Nasrallah SM, Galambos JT. Amino acid therapy of alcoholic hepatitis. Lancet 1980;2:1275–9.

[99] Simon D, Galambos JT. A randomized controlled study of peripheral parenteral nutrition in moderate and severe alcoholic hepatitis. J Hepatol 1988;7:200–7.

[100] Cabre E, Gonzalez-Huix F, Abad-Lacruz A, et al. Effect of total enteral nutrition on the short-

term outcome of severely malnourished cirrhotics: a randomized controlled trial. Gastro-enterology 1990;98:715–20.

[101] Mezey E, Caballeria J, Mitchell M, et al. Effects of parenteral amino acid supplementation on short term and long term outcomes in severe alcoholic hepatitis: a randomized controlled trial. Hepatology 1991;14:1090–6.

[102] Lesesne HR, Bozymski EM, Fallon HJ. Treatment of alcoholic hepatitis with encephalopathy: comparison of prednisolone with caloric supplements. Gastroenterology 1978;74:169–73.

[103] Galambos JT, Hersh T, Fulenwider JT, et al. Hyperalimentation in alcoholic hepatitis. Am J Gastroenterol 1979;72:535–41.

[104] Mendenhall C, Bongiovanni G, Goldberg S, et al. VA Cooperative study on alcoholic hepatitis III: changes in protein-calorie malnutrition associated with 30 days of hospitalization with and without enteral nutritional therapy. J Parenteral Enteral Nutr 1985;9:590–6.

[105] Naveau S, Pelletier G, Poynard T, et al. A randomized clinical trial of supplementary parenteral nutrion in jaundiced alcoholic cirrhotic patients. Hepatology 1986;6:270–4.

[106] Soberon S, Pauley MP, Duplantier R, et al. Metabolic effects of enteral formula feeding in alcoholic hepatitis. Hepatology 1987;7:1204–9.

[107] Kearns PJ, Young H, Garcia G, et al. Accelerated improvement of alcoholic liver disease with enteral nutrition. Gastroenterology 1992;102:200–5.

[108] Mendenhall CL, Moritz TE, Roselle GA, et al. A study of oral nutritional support with oxandrolone in a malnourished patients with alcoholic hepatitis: results of a Department of Veterans Affairs cooperative study. Hepatology 1993;17:564–76.

[109] Cabre E, Rodriguez-Iglesias P, Caballeria J, et al. Short and long-term outcome of severe alcohol-induced hepatitis treated with steroids or enteral nutrition: a multicenter randomized trial. Hepatology 2000;32:36–42.

[110] Calvey H, Davis M, Williams R. Controlled trial of nutritional supplementation, with and with-out branched chain amino acid enrichment, in treatment of acute alcoholic hepatitis. J Hepatol 1985;1:141–51.

[111] Foody W, Heuman DD, Mihas AA, et al. Nutritional therapy for alcoholic hepatitis: new life for an old idea. Gastroenterology 2001;120:1053–4.

[112] McCullough AJ, Teran JC, Bugianesi E. Guidelines for nutritional therapy in liver disease. In: Klein S, editor. The A.S.P.E.N. nutrition support practice manual. Silver Spring, MD: ASPEN Publishers; 1998. p. 1–12.

[113] Plauth M, Merli M, Kondrup J, et al. ESPEN guidelines for nutrition in liver disease and transplantation. Clin Nutr 1997;16:43–55.

[114] Florez DA, Aranda-Michel J. Nutritional management of acute and chronic liver disease. Semin Gastrointest Dis 2002;13:169–78.

[115] Saso K, Moehren G, Higashi K, et al. Differential inhibition of epidermal growth factor signaling pathways in rat hepatocytes by long-term ethanol treatment. Gastroenterology 1997; 112:2073–88.

[116] Diehl AM, Thorgeirsson SS, Steer CJ. Ethanol inhibits liver regeneration in rats without reducing transcripts of key protooncogenes. Gastroenterology 1990;99:1105–12.

[117] Fang JWS, Bird GLA, Nakamura T, et al. Hepatocyte proliferation as an indicator of outcome in acute alcoholic hepatitis. Lancet 1994;343:820–3.

[118] Black D, Lyman S, Heider TR, et al. Molecular and cellular features of hepatic regeneration. J Surg Res 2004;117:306–15.

[119] Costa RH, Kalinichenko VV, Holterman AL, et al. Transcription factor sin liver development, differentiation and regeneration. Hepatology 2003;38:1331–47.

[120] Lowes KN, Croager EJ, Olynyk JK, et al. Oval cell-mediated liver regeneration: role of cytokines and growth factors. J Gastroenterol Hepatol 2003;18:4–12.

[121] Trinchet JC, Balkau B, Poupon RE, et al. Treatment of severe alcholic hepatitis by infusion of insulin and glucagon : a multicenter sequential trial. Hepatology 1992;15:76–81.

[122] Bird G, Lau JY, Kosikinas J, et al. Insulin and glucagons infusion in acute alcoholic hepatitis: a prospective randomized controlled trial. Hepatology 1991;14:1097–101.

[123] Baker AL, Jaspan JB, Haines NW, et al. A randomized clinical trial of insulin and glucagons infusion for treatment of alcoholic hepatitis: progress report in 50 patients. Gastroenterology 1981;80:1410–4.

[124] Feher J, Cornidies A, Romany A, et al. A prospective multicenter study of insulin and glucagons infusion therapy in acute alcoholic hepatitis. J Hepatol 1987;5:224–31.

[125] Oka H, Fujiwara K, Okita K, et al. A multi-centre double blind controlled trial of glucagons and insulin therapy for severe acute hepatitis. Gastroenterol Jpn 1989;24:332–6.

[126] Berlanga J, Caballero ME, Ramirez D, et al. Epidermal growth factor protects against carbon tetrachloride-induced hepatic injury. Clin Sci (Colch) 1998;94:219–23.

[127] Cho JY, Yeon JD, Kim JY, et al. Hepatoprotection by human epidermal growth factor (hEGF) against experimental hepatitis induced by D-galactosamine (D-galN) or D-GalN/lipopolysaccharide. Biol Pharm Bull 2000;23:1243–6.

[128] Tahara M, Matsumoto K, Nukiwa T, et al. Hepatocyte growth factor leads to recovery from alcohol-induced fatty liver in rats. J Clin Invest 1999;103:313–20.

[129] Kosai K, Matsumoto K, Funakoshi H, et al. Hepatocyte growth factor prevents endotoxin-induced lethal hepatic failure in mice. Hepatology 1999;30:151–9.

[130] Hillan KJ, Logan MC, Ferrier RK, et al. Hepatocyte proliferation and serum hepatocyte growth factor levels in patients with alcoholic hepatitis. J Hepatol 1996;24:385–90.

[131] Fang JW, Bird GL, Nakamura T, et al. Hepatocyte proliferation as an indicator of outcome in acute alcoholic hepatitis. Lancet 1994;343:820–3.

[132] Takada AN, Nei J, Tamino H, et al. Effects of malotilate on ethanol-inhibited hepatocyte regeneration in rats. J Hepatol 1987;5:336–43.

[133] Hadengue A, Moreau R, Lee SS, et al. Liver hypermetabolism during alcohol withdrawal in humans. Gastroenterology 1988;94:1047–52.

[134] Hayashi N, Kasahara A, Kurosawa K, et al. Oxygen supply to the liver in patients with alcoholic liver diseases assessed by organ-reflectance spectrophotometry. Gastroenterology 1985;88:881–6.

[135] Israel Y, Kalant H, Orrego H, et al. Experimental alcohol induced hepatic necrosis: suppression by propylthiouracil. Proc Natl Acad Sci USA 1975;72:1137–41.

[136] Iturriaga H, Ugarte C, Israel Y. Hepatic vein oxygenation, liver blood flow and the rate of ethanol metabolism in recently abstinent alcoholic patients. Eur J Clin Invest 1980;10:211–8.

[137] Kasahara A, Hayashi N, Sasaki Y, et al. Hepatic circulation and hepatic oxygen consumption in alcoholic and non alcoholic fatty liver. Am J Gastroenterol 1988;83:846–9.

[138] Kessler BJ, Liebler JB, Bronfing J, et al. The hepatic blood flow and splanchnic oxygen consumption in alcoholic fatty liver. J Clin Invest 1954;33:1338–45.

[139] Israel Y, Walfish PG, Orrego H, et al. Thyroid hormones in alcoholic liver disease: effect of treatment with 6-n-propylthiouracil. Gastroenterology 1979;76:116–22.

[140] Orrego H, Kalant H, Israel Y, et al. Effect of short term therapy with PTU in patients with alcoholic liver disease. Gastroenterology 1979;76:105–15.

[141] Halle P, Pare P, Kaptein E, et al. Double-blind, controlled trial of propylthiouracil in patients with severe acute alcoholic hepatitis. Gastroenterology 1982;87:925–31.

[142] Rambaldi A, Gluud C. Meta-analysis of propylthiouracil for alcoholic liver disease—a Cochrane Hepatobiliary group review. Liver 2001;21:398–401.

[143] Rosenak BD, Moser RH, Kilgore B. Treatment of cirrhosis of the liver with testosterone propionate. Gastroenterology 1947;9:695–704.

[144] Leevy CM. Fatty liver: a study of 270 patients with biopsy proven fatty liver and a review of the literature. Medicine 1962;41:249–78.

[145] Shahidi NT. A review of the chemistry, biological action, and clinical applications of anabolic-androgenic steroids. Clin Ther 2001;23:1355–90.

[146] Orr R, Singh MF. The anabolic androgenic steroid oxandrolone in the treatment of wasting and catabolic disorders. Drugs 2004;64:725–50.

[147] Bengmark S, Olsson R. The effect of testosterone on liver healing after partial hepatectomy. Acta Chir Scand 1964;127:93–100.

[148] Maddrey WC. Is therapy with testosterone or anabolic-androgenic steroids useful in the treatment of alcoholic liver disease? Hepatology 1986;6:1033–5.

[149] Fenster LF. The nonefficacy of short term anabolic steroid therapy in alcoholic liver disease. Ann Intern Med 1966;65:738–44.

[150] Mendenhall CL, Goldberg S. Risk factors and therapy in alcoholic hepatitis (AH). Gastroenterology 1977;72:1100.

[151] Mendenhall CL, Anderson S, Garcia-Pont P, et al. Short term and long-term survival in patients with alcoholic hepatitis treated with oxandrolone and prednisolone. N Engl J Med 1984; 311:1464–70.

[152] Copenhagen Study Group for Liver Diseases. Testosterone treatment of men with alcoholic cirrhosis: a double-blind study. Hepatology 1986;6:807–13.

[153] Bonkovsky HL, Fiellin DA, Smith GS, et al. A randomized controlled trial of treatment of alcoholic hepatitis with parenteral nutrition and oxandrolone. I Short term effects on liver function. Am J Gastroenterol 1991;86:1200–8.

[154] Orr R, Singh MF. The anabolic androgenic steroid oxandrolone in the treatment of wasting and catabolic disorders: review of efficacy and safety. Drugs 2004;64:725–50.

[155] Mendenhall CL, Moritz TE, Roselle GA, et al. A study of oral nutritional support with oxandrolone in malnourished patients with alcoholic hepatitis: results of a Department of Veterans Affairs Cooperative Study. Hepatology 1993;17:564–76.

[156] Rambaldi A, Iaquinto G, Gluud C. Anabolic-androgenic steroids for alcoholic liver disease: a Cochrane review. Am J Gastroenterol 2002;97:1674–81.

[157] Poo JL, Feldmann G, Moreau A, et al. Early colchicine administration reduces hepatic fibrosis and portal hypertension in rats with bile duct ligation. J Hepatol 1993;19:90–4.

[158] Ramm GA, Powell LW, Halliday JW. Effect of colchicine on the clearance of ferritin in vivo. Am J Physiol 1990;258:G707–13.

[159] Mourelle M, Villalon C, Amezcua JL. Protective effect of colchicine on acute liver damage induced by carbon tetrachloride. J Hepatol 1988;6:337–42.

[160] Akriviadis WEA, Steindel H, Pinto PC, et al. Failure of colchicine to improve short-term survival in patients with alcoholic hepatitis. Gastroenterology 1990;99:811–8.

[161] Trinchet JC, Beaugrand M, Callard P, et al. Treatment of alcoholic hepatitis with colchicine. Results of a randomized double-blind trial. Gastroenterol Clin Biol 1989;13:551–5.

[162] Rambaldi A, Gluud C. Colchicine for alcoholic and non-alcoholic liver fibrosis or cirrhosis. Liver 2001;21:129–36.

[163] Barak AJ, Beckenhauer HC, Junnila M, et al. Dietary betaine promotes generation of hepatic S-adenosylmethionine and protects the liver from ethanol-induced fatty infiltration. Alcohol Clin Exp Res 1993;17:552–5.

[164] Lieber CS, Casini A, DeCarli LM, et al. S-adenosyl-L-methionine attenuates alcohol-induced liver injury in the baboon. Hepatology 1990;11:165–72.

[165] Lieber CS, Robins SJ, Li J, et al. Phosphatidylcholine protects against fibrosis and cirrhosis in the baboon. Gastroenterology 1994;106:152–9.

[166] McClain CJ, Hill DB, Song Z, et al. S-Adenosymethionine, cytokines, and alcoholic liver disease. Alcohol 2002;27:185–92.

[167] Purohit V, Russo D. Role of S-adenosyl L methionine in the treatment of alcoholic liver disease: introduction and summary of the symposium. Alcohol 2002;27:151–4.

[168] Lee TD, Sadda MR, Mendler MH, et al. Abnormal hepatic methionine and glutathione metabolism in patients with alcoholic hepatitis. Alcohol Clin Exp Res 2004;28:173–81.

[169] Mato JM, Camara J, Fernandez de Paz J, et al. S-Adenosylmethionine in alcoholic liver cirrhosis: a randomized placebo-controlled double blind multicenter clinical trial. J Hepatol 1999;30:1081–9.

[170] Rambaldi A, Gluud C. S-adenosyl-L-methionine for alcoholic liver disease. Cochrane Database Syst Rev 2004;3.

[171] Lieber CS. A-Adenosyl-L-methionine and alcoholic liver disease in animal models: implications for early intervention in human beings. Alcohol 2002;27:173–7.

[172] Thomas CE, Reed DJ. Current status of calcium in hepatocyte injury. Hepatalogy 1989;10: 375–84.

[173] Takei Y, Marzi I, Kauffman FC, et al. Prevention of early graft failure by the calcium channel blocker nisoldipine: involvement of Kupffer cells. Transplantation 1990;50:14–20.

[174] Imuro Y, Ikejima K, Rose ML, et al. Niodipine, a dihydopyridine type calcium channel blocker, prevents alcoholic hepatitis caused by chronic intragastric ethanol exposure in the rat. Hepatology 1996;24:391–7.

[175] Bird GLA, Prach AT, McMahon AD, et al. Randomized controlled double-blind trial of the calcium channel antagonist amlodipine in the treatment of acute alcoholic hepatitis. J Hepatol 1998;28:194–8.

[176] Mezey E. Prevention of alcohol-induced hepatic fibrosis by phosphatidylcholine. Gastroenterology 1994;106:257–9.

[177] Lieber CS, Casini A, DeCarli LM, et al. Attenuation of alcohol-induced hepatic fibrosis by polyunsaturated lecithin. Hepatology 1990;12:1390–8.

[178] Lieber CS, Casini A, DeCarli LM, et al. S-Adenosyl-L-methionine attenuates alcohol-induced liver injury in the baboon. Hepatology 1990;11:165–72.

[179] Lieber CS, Leo MA, Aleynik SI, et al. Polyenylphospatidylcholine decreases alcohol-induced oxidative stress in the baboon. Alcohol Clin Exp Res 1997;21:375–9.

[180] Aleynik SI, Lieber CS. Polyenylphospatidylcholine corrects the alcohol-induced hepatic oxidative stress by restoring S-adenosylmethionine. Alcohol Alcohol 2003;38:208–12.

[181] Lieber CS, Weiss DG, Groszmann R, et al, for the Veterans Affairs Cooperative Study 391 Group II. Veterans Affairs Cooperative Study of polyenylphosphatidylcholine in alcoholic liver disease. Alcohol Clin Exp Res 2003;27:1765–72.

[182] Seeff LB, Lindsay KL, Bacon BR, et al. Complementary and alternative medicine in chronic liver disease. Hepatology 2003;34:595–603.

[183] Berger J, Kowdley KV. Is silymarin hepatoprotective in alcoholic liver disease? J Clin Gastroenterol 2003;37:278–9.

[184] Saller R, Meier R, Brignoli R. The use of silymarin in the treatment of liver diseases. Drugs 2001;61:2035–63.

[185] Lieber CS, Leo MA, Cao Q, et al. Silymarin retards the progression of alcohol-induced hepatic fibrosis in baboons. J Clin Gastroenterol 2003;37:336–9.

[186] Pares A, Planas R, Torres M, et al. Effects of silymarin in alcoholic patients with cirrhosis of the liver: results of a controlled, double-blind, randomized and multicenter trial. J Hepatol 1998;28:615–21.

[187] Trinchet JC, Coste T, Levy VG, et al. Treatment of alcoholic hepatitis with silymarin. A double-blind comparative study in 116 patients. Gastroenterol Clin Biol 1989;13:120–4.

[188] Harrison SA, Torgerson S, Hayashi P, et al. Vitamin E and vitamin C treatment improves fibrosis in patients with nonalcoholic steatohepatitis. Am J Gastroenterol 2003;98:2485–90.

[189] Mezey E, Potter JJ, Rennie-Tankersley L, et al. A randomized placebo controlled trial of vitamin E for alcoholic hepatitis. J Hepatol 2004;40:40–6.

[190] Jalan R, Sen S, Steiner C, et al. Extracorporeal liver support with molecular adsorbents recirculating system in patients with severe acute alcoholic hepatitis. J Hepatol 2003;38:24–31.

[191] Tsuji Y, Kumashiro R, Ishil K, et al. Severe alcoholic hepatitis successfully treated by leukocytapharesis: a case report. Alcohol Clin Exp Res 2003;27:26S–31S.

[192] Shakil AO, Pinna A, Demetris J, et al. Survival and quality of life after liver transplantation for acute alcoholic hepatitis. Liver Transplant Surg 1997;3:240–4.

[193] Mutimer DJ, Burra P, Neuberger JM, et al. Managing severe alcoholic hepatitis complicated by renal failure. Q J Med 1993;86:649–56.

[194] Tome S, Martinez-Rey C, Gonzalez-Quintela A, et al. Influence of superimposed alcoholic hepatitis on the outcome of liver transplantation for end-stage alcoholic liver disease. J Hepatol 2002;36:793–8.

[195] Lucey MR. Is liver transplantation an appropriate treatment for acute alcoholic hepatitis? J Hepatol 2002;36:829–31.

[196] Jiminez JL, Punzon C, Navarro J, et al. Phospodiesterase 4 inhibitors prevent cytokine secretion by T lymphocytes by inhibiting nuclear factor κB and nuclear factor of activated T cells activation. J Pharmacol Exp Ther 2001;299:753–9.

[197] Sanchez S, Albornoz L, Bandi JC, et al. Pentoxifylline, a drug with rheological effects, decreases portal pressure in an experimental model of cirrhosis. Eur J Gastroenterol Hepatol 1997;9:27–31.

[198] Soupison T, Yang S, Bernard C, et al. Acute haemodynamic responses and inhibition of tumour necrosis factor-alpha by pentoxifylline in rats with cirrhosis. Clin Sci (Colch) 1996;91: 29–33.

[199] Akrivadis E, Botla R, Briggs W, et al. Pentoxifylline improves short-term survival in severe acute alcoholic hepatitis: a double-blind, placebo-controlled trial. Gastroenterology 2000;119: 1637–48.

[200] Spahr L, Rubbia-Brandt L, Frossard JK, et al. Combination of steroids with infliximab or placebo in severe alcoholic hepatitis: a randomized controlled pilot study. J Hepatol 2002; 37:448–55.

[201] Tilg H, Jalan R, Kaser A, et al. Anti-tumor necrosis factor-alpha monoclonal antibody therapy in severe alcoholic hepatitis. J Hepatol 2003;38:419–25.

[202] Fong TL, Tran T. Open label pilot study of the effects of a chimeric anti-tumor necrosis factor monoclonal antibody in patients with severe acute alcoholic hepatitis. Hepatology 2001;A2105:A698.

[203] Naveau S, Chollet-Martin S, Dharancy S, et al. A double blind randomized controlled trial of infliximab associated with prednisolone in acute alcoholic hepatitis. Gastroenterology 2004; 126:S1137.

[204] Naveau S, Chollet-Martin S, Dharancy S, et al. A double-blind randomized controlled trial of infliximab associated with prednisolone in acute alcoholic hepatitis. Hepatology 2004;39: 1390–7.

[205] McClain CJ, Hill DB, Barve SS. Infliximab and prednisolone: too much of a good thing? Hepatology 2004;39:1488–90.

[206] Akerman PA, Cote PM, Yang MQ, et al. Long-term ethanol consumption alters the hepatic response to the regenerative effects of tumour necrosis factor-alpha. Hepatology 1993;17: 1066–73.

[207] Menon KV, Stadheim L, Kamath PS, et al. A pilot study of the safety and tolerability of etanercept in patients with alcoholic hepatitis. Am J Gastroenterol 2004;99:255–60.

[208] Ziol M, Tepper M, Loherz M, et al. Clinical and biological relevance of hepatocyte apoptosis in alcoholic hepatitis. J Hepatol 2001;34:254–60.

[209] Natori S, Rust C, Stadheim LM, et al. Hepatocyte apoptosis is a pathologic feature of human alcoholic hepatitis. J Hepatol 2001;34:248–53.

[210] Day CP. Apoptosis in alcoholic hepatitis: a novel therapeutic target? J Hepatol 2001;34:330–3.

ELSEVIER
SAUNDERS

CLINICS IN
LIVER DISEASE

Clin Liver Dis 9 (2005) 135–149

Long-term Management of Alcoholic Liver Disease

Jamilé Wakim-Fleming, MD*, Kevin D. Mullen, MD

Case Western Reserve School of Medicine, 2580 Metrohealth Drive, Room G-632A, Cleveland, OH 44109, USA

Alcohol is the most common recreational drug ingested by Americans and Northern Europeans. Even though alcohol consumption in the United States has been declining since the 1980s, 14 million people still meet criteria for alcoholism. Two million are suspected of having liver disease. Nearly 100,000 alcohol-related deaths occur each year in the United States, and 14,000 people die of cirrhosis [1].

There is a direct correlation between alcohol consumption and liver-related mortality [2]. It is estimated that men who drink regularly and for many years an amount of ethanol that is more than 80 g/d (eight 12-oz servings of beer at 4.5%, 1~L of wine at 4.5%, or 0.5 pint of distilled spirits) will be at substantial risk of developing clinical liver disease [3]. Women who drink the same amount are two to four times more likely than men to develop alcoholic liver disease (ALD), and they exhibit a tendency to disease progression even with abstinence [4–6].

The ceiling for low-risk alcohol use advocated in the US government is one standard drink a day for women and two a day for men. Because of the physiologic changes that occur with aging, the National Institute on Alcohol Abuse and Alcoholism recommends that men and women over 65 years of age do not consume more than one drink a day [7]. A standard drink is defined as 12 g of alcohol or one 12-oz bottle of beer (4.5%) or one 5-oz glass of wine (12.9%) or 1.5 oz of 80-proof distilled spirits [6].

The liver is the primary site of ethanol metabolism. The liver cell contains the largest amount of enzymes involved in the metabolism of ethanol. Hepatic damage or alcohol liver disease has been recognized for centuries as the hall-

---

* Corresponding author.
E-mail addresses: jwfleming@metrohealth.org, FLEMINJ1@CCF.ORG (J. Wakim-Fleming).

mark of chronic alcohol ingestion. Only a small proportion of alcoholic patients develop liver damage. This is partly due to genetic or hereditary predisposition, female gender, obesity, and other factors including hepatitis C virus coinfection [8].

Alcoholism is the most common cause of cirrhosis in the United States.

ALD encompasses a spectrum of three main, often overlapping, histologic features: steatosis, acute alcoholic hepatitis, and cirrhosis.

Abstinence often reverses the steatosis or fatty infiltration. Alcoholic hepatitis is more severe; patients are symptomatic, and often require admission to the hospital. If patients continue to drink, up to 80% may develop cirrhosis. Once cirrhosis develops, abstinence of alcohol may reverse the coexisting features of steatosis or fibrosis but not cirrhosis.

There is continuous debate over the reversibility of cirrhosis and fibrosis. When fibrous septa carrying shunting vessels extend through the parenchyma and reach central and portal tracts forming anastomosis between draining vessels and causing architectural distortion, then full-blown cirrhosis is considered to be present. Studies have shown that lesser degrees of fibrosis are reversible, and even early cirrhosis is. The continuous damage to liver cells with the continued ingestion of ethanol may lead to an irreversible stage of cirrhosis and its morbidity and mortality [9,10].

Risk factors for fibrosis after adjusting for daily alcohol intake and total duration of alcohol abuse were noted to be: body mass index, iron overload assessed by Perl's stain, and elevated blood glucose level [11].

Alcohol is a procarcinogen. The mechanism is multifactorial: some of these factors include a direct toxic effect on hepatocytes with DNA hypomethylation, lipid peroxidation, activation of Kupffer cells, and induction of CYP2E1 with release of reactive oxidant species, tumor necrosis factor alpha, and other procarcinogenic substances [12]. Cirrhosis of the liver is almost always present in alcoholic livers that go on to develop hepatocellular carcinoma. The associated viral infection with hepatitis B and hepatitis C further increases the risk of hepatocellular carcinoma [13].

Overview of management

The management of patients with alcoholic cirrhosis is similar in many ways to the management of patients with cirrhosis of other etiologies. However, because of the nature of the different pathophysiologic mechanisms related to alcohol toxicity, subtle nuances in the management of alcoholics may exist, and these are addressed in this article.

Abstinence is the cornerstone of therapy. Its beneficial effects are notable before and after liver transplantation. Alcohol not only affects the liver but other organs in the body, worsening morbidity and mortality. The effects of abstinence were observed in clinical, endoscopic, and hemodynamic parameters, with improved survival and a decreased probability for bleeding.

Brief interventions to educate and inform patients about the consequences of their drinking habit and to guide and advise them to change their behavior have shown to significantly increase the chances of moderating the amount of ethanol ingestion by these patients [14]. These methods have also shown to be cost effective [15]. In a randomized controlled trial, alcohol-dependent patients were given a manual-guided psychologic treatment that included cognitive–behavioral therapy and motivation enhancement therapy. These patients were compared with a group of patients who did not receive the manuals. Patients who received the manuals and followed the treatment guidelines had reduced the amount of ingested ethanol compared with those patients who did not receive the treatment guide [16].

Therefore, emphasis on abstinence via collaborative work of physicians and health care providers is possible and crucial in arresting the progression of liver disease, and it cannot be overstated. Abstinence is important in the initial management of ALD as well as when cirrhosis develops. In patients with established cirrhosis, abstinence may help identify and prevent early complications and mortality related to the cirrhosis.

Other important elements in the management of ALD include identification and exclusion of other associated causes of liver injury, correction of nutritional deficiencies, prevention and treatment of complications of cirrhosis, and referral to liver transplantation when medical treatment fails.

Long-term complications and management

Esophageal varices

In 1988, Practice Guidelines for the treatment of portal hypertension recommended screening for esophageal varices in all patients with cirrhosis Child B and C, and for child A, who have low platelet counts < 140,000, enlarged portal vein diameter > 13 mm, or evidence of collateral circulation on liver Doppler ultrasound. Patients who have no varices on screening upper endoscopy (EGD), should undergo repeat EGD every 2 years or every year if liver function deteriorates. Patients who had small varices on screening EGD should undergo a repeat EGD in a year and treatment with a nonselective beta-blocker should be started for the prevention of first variceal bleeding [17]. A recent study suggests that primary prophylaxis with a beta-blocker (Nadolol) in alcoholic and nonalcoholic patients with compensated cirrhosis and small esophageal varices may prevent growth in the size of the varices over time [18].

It is known that when patients abstain from alcohol consumption, their varices may regress [19,20]. Continued alcohol consumption is a risk factor for late variceal bleeding that is > 6 weeks after the initial bleeding episode, and the cumulative probability of survival is greater for abstainers than for nonabstainers $P < 0.05$ [21,22].

Ascites

Alcohol-induced liver injury may lead to sinusoidal and presinusoidal portal hypertension. Ascites is characterized by an elevated serum-ascites albumin gradient (SAAG) level greater than 1.1. It is advisable to verify that SAAG is >1.1. If not, other causes of ascites should be considered. As in ascites due to other causes of liver injury, diuretics and salt restriction are first-line therapy, and are most likely to induce a clinical response. It is important to treat the underlying liver disease in the setting of portal hypertension, and more specifically, to convince the patient to stop drinking. It is thought that ascites may resolve or become more responsive to medical therapy with abstinence and time [23]. In an article by Vorobioff, ascites was noted to be present in most patients who continued to drink alcohol compared with those who were abstinent ($P < 0.01$) [22].

Hematologic effects

Cirrhosis due to alcohol consumption is associated with leukopenia, thrombocytopenia, low hemoglobin levels, and increased mean corpuscular volume (MCV) and mean corpuscular hemoglobin (MCH). Despite the peripheral cytopenia, the bone marrow may be hypercellular and rich in adipocytes [24–26].

Continuous heavy alcohol ingestion may worsen anemia. Anemia may be myelodysplastic, sideroblastic, or hemolytic secondary to membrane defect (spur cells) induced by alcoholism and pyridoxine/B_{12}/riboflavin deficiencies [24,25, 27–29]. Other proposed mechanisms of anemia include agglutination of a soluble variant of the human asialoglycoprotein receptor causing mechanical shear stress on the red cells [30].

Splenomegaly, deficiency of vitamin K, and thrombocytopenia singly and in concert can contribute to hemostatic deficiencies in patients with long-standing ALD.

Hepatorenal syndrome

Aggravation of the underlying ALD by continuous alcohol ingestion is the most common predisposing factor for hepatorenal syndrome (HRS) [31].

When HRS develops in the setting of alcoholic cirrhosis, its treatment is not different from the treatment of HRS in nonalcoholic cirrhosis. Vasoconstrictive agents such as terlipressin and midodrine, and a transjugular intrahepatic portosystemic shunt (TIPS) may be effective in improving kidney function. Liver transplantation remains the best option in patients without contraindication to the procedure because the outcome of HRS remains poor [32,33].

Albumin infusion and antibiotic therapy for patients with spontaneous bacterial peritonitis have shown to reduce the incidence of renal impairment; hence HRS and death in comparison with treatment with antibiotic alone [34]. Randomized controlled trials suggest that pentoxifyline decreases mortality in patients with acute alcoholic hepatitis primarily by preventing the development of HRS [32].

Hepatic osteodystophy

Alcohol can directly induce adipogenesis, decrease osteogenesis and osteogenic differentiation, and produce intracellular lipid deposits resulting in necrosis and death of osteocytes [26,35].

Chronic alcohol ingestion has a direct effect on osteoblast formation, and could cause osteoporosis and fractures [36,37]. Peris demonstrated that chronic alcoholics frequently have bone loss at the lumbar spine and at the femoral neck related to the duration of alcohol intake. Low levels of vitamin D supports its role in the development of osteopenia in chronic alcoholism [38]. Patients at risk for osteoporosis should undergo bone densitometry screening, and appropriate treatment should be initiated if necessary [39,40].

Portopulmonary hypertension and hepatopulmonary syndrome

Portopulmonary hypertension (PPHTN) and hepatopulmonary syndrome (HPS) occur in cirrhotic and noncirrhotic individuals with spontaneous portosystemic shunts. There is no specific etiology for the cirrhosis that is associated with a higher risk for developing HPS or PPHTN. Medical therapy is ineffective for hepatopulmonary syndrome, but liver transplantation is curative. Intravenous prostacycline is the agent of choice for portopulmonary hypertension [41].

Disorders in endocrine function

The prevalence of impotence is increased in males who chronically abuse alcohol [42]. This may be due to the direct effect of ethanol at inducing primary hypogonadism as well as hypothalamic–pituitary inhibition. Men with alcoholic cirrhosis may show signs of feminization related to increased peripheral conversion of androgens. In men who abstain from alcohol, a spontaneous recovery of sexual function can occur, especially when no testicular atrophy is present and when the response of gonadotrophins to luteinizing hormone-releasing hormone (LH-RH) stimulation is normal. Therapeutically, only the administration of nonaromatizable androgens in high doses seems to lead to recovery of potency [43,44].

When 60 chronic alcoholic and impotent men who stopped ingesting ethanol were followed, 25% of them recovered their sexual function spontaneously. Those not recovering spontaneously were treated sequentially with clomiphene, human chorionic gonadotropin, and an oral exogenous androgen. Only the treatment with androgen produced acceptable results but at unusually high doses, suggesting the possibility of androgen insensitivity in such men [45]. Others have shown that impotence results from impaired testicular androgenic secretion by the action of alcohol or its metabolite, acetaldehyde [43].

End-stage liver disease may be associated with the euthyroid sick state. Cirrhosis related to alcohol and hepatitis C may increase the risk of developing diabetes mellitus [46].

Hepatic encephalopathy

Hepatic encephalopathy (HE) tends to present in patients with alcoholic cirrhosis when signs of portal hypertension and loss of synthetic liver function are obvious. In contrast, patients with liver disease who progress at a slower rate are inclined to present with bouts of HE before loss of liver function is obvious. Correction of the underlying precipitating agents is important in possibly reversing the encephalopathy [47,48].

The long-term care of patients with alcohol-induced cirrhosis should always be vigilant in regard to the development of HE. Generally, this complication starts to appear when substantial loss of liver synthetic function is noted. When major portosystemic shunting of blood is superimposed on chronic cirrhosis, HE may start to become a major management issue [48,49]. This is seen in an accelerated fashion after the creation of a TIPS for control of recurrent variceal bleeding. Both the shunt itself and the portoprivic hepatic perfusion contribute to this phenomenon [48,49]. About 20% to 25% of patients will develop bouts of overt HE after TIPS placement [50]. Usually, unless liver function deteriorates significantly, this tendency to develop HE is self-limited with the standard bare stents. The newer covered stents may be associated with more persistent HE because those stents do not gradually close or narrow over time [51,52]. Critical factors determining HE after TIPS appear to be: (1) underlying liver function, (2) age of the patient, (3) diameter of the stent, and (4) the poststent insertion residual portal pressure [50].

The other instance of development of HE in alcoholic cirrhotics who still have relatively well-preserved hepatic synthetic function (ie, albumin >3.0 g, prothrombin time <3 seconds prolonged) is the formation of huge portovenous collateral vessels. These may occur anywhere the portal and venous systems are in contact, but most often occur in the splenorenal region. Any patients with bouts of HE and preserved liver function should be carefully managed to identify these large collaterals because they can be amenable to radiologic therapy. Although the collaterals never develop to the degree of normalizing portal pressure, they do tend to be associated with small or absent varices and little ascites. Successful identification of these types of vessels can lead to an attempt at their closure. This would completely abolish the tendency to develop HE [53].

Another aspect of HE in long-standing alcoholic cirrhotics is what we now term "minimal encephalopathy." Formerly, this used to be called subclinical HE [47,54]. There is some evidence to suggest that quality of life may be reduced in patients with minimal encephalopathy [47,55], although there is still a bit of disagreement about its effect on driving ability [56,57]. It is uncertain if treatment with lactulose improves this situation. The recent report that detection of minimal HE with psychometric testing predicts subsequent bouts of HE raises the issue that prophylactic treatment might postpone the development of overt HE [47,58].

The treatment of HE is well standardized if somewhat unproven in today's exacting evidence-based medicine. Protein restriction generally seems to be justifiably waning as a treatment for HE [59,60]. Some suggest that protein intake may have a limited role in precipitating encephalopathy, whereas suppressing protein breakdown may be more effective. Supplementing patients who have HE and malnutrition with branched chain amino acids may achieve a positive nitrogen balance without precipitating HE [61,62]. Vegetable diets have been noted to improve HE because they are less ammoniogenic, provide an increased amount of fiber, and increase elimination and incorporation of nitrogen in fecal bacteria [63]. Otherwise, treatment of overt HE in alcoholic cirrhotics is not appreciably different than in other forms of cirrhosis except for one part, that is, demanding prolonged sobriety and active participation in detoxification programs. This may preclude some alcoholic cirrhotics from qualifying for a liver transplant if the assessment process starts after HE has become a clinical problem. Some patients cannot complete alcohol rehabilitation programs because of frequent bouts of HE. Accordingly, getting those issues sorted out before HE appears is important.

Liver transplantation remains the only option for truly intractable HE [48].

Pharmacologic therapy

Ursodeoxycholic acid

Ursodeoxycholic acid is a tertiary hydrophilic bile acid that has been used in the management of cholestatic liver diseases. Its mechanism of action is to displace toxic bile and protect hepatocytes and bile duct cells from injury caused by bile acids and alcohol. In a multicenter double-blind controlled trial of patients with alcoholic cirrhosis and jaundice, the administration of ursodeoxycholic acid at 13 to 15 mg/kg/d did not show a survival benefit at 6-month follow-up of patients with severe alcohol-induced cirrhosis [64].

Anabolic steroids

Using the Cochrane Database, only randomized clinical trials studying patients with alcoholic steatosis, alcoholic fibrosis, alcoholic hepatitis, or alcoholic cirrhosis were included. Interventions encompassed anabolic–androgenic steroids at any dose or duration versus placebo or no intervention. Anabolic–androgenic steroids did not demonstrate any significant beneficial effects on any clinically important outcomes (mortality, liver-related mortality, liver complications, and histology) of patients with ALD [65]. Thus, androgenic steroids are not approved by the US Food and Drug Administration in the treatment of such patients.

Propylthiouracil

Six randomized clinical trials have addressed the question of whether propylthiouracil has any efficacy in patients with ALD. Interventions encompassed propylthiouracil at any dose versus placebo or no intervention. This systematic review could not demonstrate any significant efficacy of propylthiouracil on any clinically important outcomes (mortality, liver-related mortality, liver complications, and liver histology) of patients with ALD. Propylthiouracil was associated with adverse events, and there is no evidence for using it in the management of ALD outside randomized clinical trials [66].

Colchicine

Colchicine is an antiinflammatory and antifibrotic drug. A long-term, randomized, double-blind, placebo-controlled trial was conducted to evaluate the efficacy of colchicine in alcoholic cirrhosis biopsy proven. Colchicine did not appear to overcome the progression and natural history of long-established alcoholic cirrhosis [67].

Another study combining the results of 14 randomized clinical trials including 1138 patients demonstrated no significant effects of colchicine on mortality, liver-related mortality, or complications. Colchicine was associated with a significantly increased risk of adverse events. The conclusion was that colchicine should not be used for liver fibrosis or liver cirrhosis irrespective of etiology [68].

Silymarin

Silymarin is an antioxidant derived from the milk thistle plant. It increases superoxide dismutase (SOD) activity of lymphocytes and erythrocytes, as well as the expression of SOD in lymphocytes. Silymarin has also been shown to increase patient serum levels of glutathione.

Studies are inconsistent in regard to the effects of silymarin therapy in patients with alcoholic cirrhosis. For instance, a study by Ferenci and colleagues [69] showed a significant survival benefit of patients with cirrhosis Child-Pugh class A treated with silymarin compared with patients given placebo. The 4-year survival rate was $58\% \pm 9\%$ in Silymarin-treated patients and $39\% \pm 9\%$ in the placebo group ($P = 0.036$). Analysis of subgroups indicated that treatment was effective in patients with alcoholic cirrhosis ($P = 0.01$) and in patients initially rated "Child A" cirrhosis ($P = 0.03$). No side effects of drug treatment were observed. The study by Wellington is a randomized, double-blind trial of patients with alcoholic cirrhosis treated with silymarin at a dose of 420 mg/d. Silmaryn improved liver function tests (aspartate aminotransferase, alanine aminotransferase, gamma-glutamyltransferase, and bilirubin) in the group with alcoholic cirrhosis but not in the group with viral hepatitis [70]. In a controlled double-blinded randomized multicenter trial, silymarin did not demonstrate an effect on survival in alcoholic patients with liver cirrhosis [71]. Therefore, silymarin could not be recommended in the management of patients with alcohol-induced liver disease.

S adenosyl methionine

Alcohol blocks the formation of glutathione from methionine by blocking the enzyme M acetyl transferase. Glutathione is the major antioxidant of the liver cell. Randomized controlled trials did not show significant effects of S adenosyl methionine (SAMe) on mortality, liver-related mortality, or transplantation. Thus, SAMe is not recommended in the management of ALD [72,73].

Nutrition and immunity in alcoholic cirrhotics

Malnutrition is common in patients with chronic liver disease and in patients with cirrhosis regardless of its etiology. Malnutrition hastens disease progression and mortality. The decrease in caloric intake seems to be an independent risk factor of short-term mortality in hospitalized cirrhotic patients [74].

Liver cirrhosis in the advanced stage is characterized by protein wasting, muscle mass loss, hypoalbuminemia, and abnormal aminoacid metabolism [75]. Some studies have shown that muscle strength is substantially weakened in patients with liver cirrhosis related to alcohol. This was related to the degree of malnutrition, but not to the severity of liver disease, neuropathy, or duration of abstinence from ethanol ingestion [76].

Malnutrition is more severe in alcoholics of lower social economic class due to poor nutritional intake and chronic alcohol intake. The consequence is a vicious circle and a poor outcome. Cirrhotic malnourished people are more likely to present with infectious complications and immunologic deficiencies. Alcohol per se suppresses the immune system via several mechanisms. It induces secretion of glucocorticoids by the adrenals via the hypothalamic /pituitary axis, decreases estrogen production in women, impairs chemotaxis, and alters the production of macrophages and cytokines [77–80].

Nutritional support has shown to improve malnutrition-related complications such as reduced cell-mediated immunity [70,81].

Therefore, malnourished alcoholics should be offered adequate nutritional support either enterally or parenterally [47]. Micronutrient deficiencies of thiamine and folate typically encountered in alcoholics should be replenished, especially in the setting of encephalopathy due to Wernicke and Korsakoff syndromes. Fat-soluble vitamin deficiencies should also be replenished.

In one study spironolactone-treated alcoholic cirrhotic patients had less pronounced muscle weakness in comparison to those who did not receive spironolactone [82].

Assessing surgical risks in alcoholic cirrhotics

When assessing patients with liver disease for candidacy for surgery, several factors need to be considered: (1) signs and symptoms, (2) coagulopathy, (3) biochemical evidence of liver disease, (4) the type of anesthetics to be used, (5) the overall physical condition and nutritional status of the patient, and (6) the type of surgery and its urgency.

An elective surgery performed on patients with decompensated liver disease carries a high surgical risk. In general, patients with good synthetic liver function and Child-Pugh class A do well compared with patients with jaundice, ascites, and decompensated liver.

Patients with alcoholic cirrhosis may have nutritional deficiencies in addition to other organ damage that will complicate their postoperative course. Therefore, nutritional and systemic supports are required perioperatively.

Drug toxicity in alcoholic cirrhotics

Alcoholic cirrhotics are more susceptible to acetaminophen toxicity in the presence of continuous ethanol ingestion. In general, patients with advanced stages of cirrhosis should avoid nonsteroidal anti-inflammatory drugs, aminoglycosides, ACE inhibitors, and beta-lactam antibiotics, which may cause hypoprothrombinemia related to inhibition of synthesis of vitamin K-dependent clotting factors [83].

Prevention

Screening for hepatocellular carcinoma

Screening with serial serum alpha-fetoprotein measurement combined with ultrasound examination of the liver has become a standard of practice for cirrhotic patients regardless of the etiology of cirrhosis [84]. This method was approved at the Barcelona-2000 European Association for the Study of the Liver conference [85].

These tests are poorly sensitive and specific, and there are no randomized controlled trials addressing the benefits of screening in cirrhotic patients.

Recommendations for viral hepatitis surveillance

Both the National Institutes of Health (NIH) and the Centers for Disease Control and Prevention (CDC) recommend vaccinating all patients with chronic liver disease against viral hepatitis A infection. The NIH recommends vaccinating hepatitis C patients against hepatitis B infection. The CDC recommends vaccinating all patients with chronic liver disease at risk for hepatitis B infection against hepatitis B infection (www.cdc.gov.recommend) [86].

Surveillance for esophageal varices

This topic was discussed earlier in "Long-term complications and management."

Liver transplantation

The survival of patients after liver transplant secondary to alcoholic cirrhosis parallels that of patients with cirrhosis due to other causes [87,88]. Considering this successful outcome, liver transplantation has been performed in increasing numbers in this group of patients [89].

Timing of the transplantation remains an issue. Six months of abstinence from alcohol is a common criterion for liver transplantation eligibility. However, this 6-month rule did not seem to predict relapse after transplantation, and there is controversy about whether this rule should be strictly applied [90]. A family history of alcoholism seems to be an independent predictor of alcohol relapse after liver transplantation [91]. One study showed that 10% to 20% of alcoholics relapse after liver transplantation; survival was not affected after 53 months of follow-up, but their grafts were injured from poor compliance with immunosuppressive drugs and alcohol-related transplant injury [64].

A multidisciplinary approach that enhances the interaction between the patient and the transplant team seems to help sustain sobriety before and after liver transplantation [92].

Significant irreversible brain damage contraindicates liver transplantation. Autonomic dysfunction will most likely improve after transplantation [93].

References

[1] Maher JJ. Alcoholic liver disease. In: Feldman M, Sleisenger M, Fordtran J, editors. Gastrointestinal and liver disease. Philadelphia: Elsevier; 2002. p. 1375–91.

[2] Ramstedt M. Per capita alcohol consumption and liver cirrhosis mortality in 14 European countries. Addiction 2001;96(Suppl 1):S19–33.

[3] Marbet UA, Bianchi L, Meury U, et al. Long-term histological evaluation of the natural history and prognostic factors of alcoholic liver disease. J Hepatol 1987;4(3):364–72.

[4] Pares A, Caballeria J, Bruguera M, et al. Histological course of alcoholic hepatitis. influence of abstinence, sex and extent of hepatic damage. J Hepatol 1986;2(1):33–42.

[5] Moshage H. Alcoholic liver disease: a matter of hormones? J Hepatol 2001;35(1):130–3.

[6] Becker U, Deis A, Sorensen TI, et al. Prediction of risk of liver disease by alcohol intake, sex, and age: a prospective population study. Hepatology 1996;23(5):1025–9.

[7] 10th special report to the US Congress on alcohol and health: highlights from current research from the Secretary of Health and Human Services. US Department of Health and Human Services, Public Health Service, National Institutes of Health, National Institute on Alcohol

Abuse and Alcoholism. NIH publication no. 00-1583. Bethesda (MD): National Institutes of Health; 2000. p. 429–30.

[8] McCullough AJ, O'Connor JF. Alcoholic liver disease: proposed recommendations for the American College of Gastroenterology. Am J Gastroenterol 1998;93(11):2022–36.

[9] Friedman SL. Liver fibrosis—from bench to bedside. J Hepatol 2003;38(Suppl 1):S38–53.

[10] Desmet VJ, Roskams T. Cirrhosis reversal: a duel between dogma and myth. J Hepatol 2004; 40(5):860–7.

[11] Raynard B, Balian A, Fallik D, et al. Risk factors of fibrosis in alcohol-induced liver disease. Hepatology 2002;35(3):635–8.

[12] Tavill AS, Qadri AM. Alcohol and iron. Semin Liver Dis 2004;24(3):317–25.

[13] Stickel F, Schuppan D, Hahn EG, et al. Cocarcinogenic effects of alcohol in hepatocarcinogenesis. Gut 2002;51(1):132–9.

[14] Kadden RM. Project MATCH: treatment main effects and matching results. Alcohol Clin Exp Res 1996;20(8 Suppl):196A–7A.

[15] Fleming MF, Mundt MP, French MT, et al. Benefit-cost analysis of brief physician advice with problem drinkers in primary care settings. Med Care 2000;38(1):7–18.

[16] Wilk AI, Jensen NM, Havighurst TC. Meta-analysis of randomized control trials addressing brief interventions in heavy alcohol drinkers. J Gen Intern Med 1997;12(5):274–83.

[17] Grace ND, Groszmann RJ, Garcia-Tsao G, et al. Portal hypertension and variceal bleeding: an AASLD single topic symposium. Hepatology 1998;28(3):868–80.

[18] Merkel C, Marin R, Angeli P, et al. A placebo-controlled clinical trial of nadolol in the prophylaxis of growth of small esophageal varices in cirrhosis. Gastroenterology 2004;127(2): 476–84.

[19] Baker LA, Smith C, Lieberman G. The natural history of esophageal varices; a study of 115 cirrhotic patients in whom varices were diagnosed prior to bleeding. Am J Med 1959;26(2): 228–37.

[20] Dagradi AE. The natural history of esophageal varices in patients with alcoholic liver cirrhosis. An endoscopic and clinical study. Am J Gastroenterol 1972;57(6):520–40.

[21] de Franchis R, Primignani M. Why do varices bleed? Gastroenterol Clin North Am 1992; 21(1):85–101.

[22] Vorobioff J, Groszmann RJ, Picabea E, et al. Prognostic value of hepatic venous pressure gradient measurements in alcoholic cirrhosis: a 10-year prospective study. Gastroenterology 1996; 111(3):701–9.

[23] Runyon BA. Management of adult patients with ascites due to cirrhosis. Hepatology 2004; 39(3):841–56.

[24] Michot F, Gut J. Alcohol-induced bone marrow damage. A bone marrow study in alcohol-dependent individuals. Acta Haematol 1987;78(4):252–7.

[25] Batista JN, Santolaria F, Gonzalez-Reimers E, et al. Evaluation of marrow cellularity in alcoholism and hepatic cirrhosis, by aspiration, biopsy and histomorphometric. Drug Alcohol Depend 1988;22(1–2):27–31.

[26] Wezeman FH, Gong Z. Adipogenic effect of alcohol on human bone marrow-derived mesenchymal stem cells. Alcohol Clin Exp Res 2004;28(7):1091–101.

[27] Lieber CS. Hepatic, metabolic and toxic effects of ethanol: 1991 update. Alcohol Clin Exp Res 1991;15(4):573–92.

[28] Lieber CS. Alcoholic liver injury: pathogenesis and therapy in 2001. Pathol Biol [Paris] 2001; 49(9):738–52.

[29] Ishak KG, Zimmerman HJ, Ray MB. Alcoholic liver disease: pathologic, pathogenetic and clinical aspects. Alcohol Clin Exp Res 1991;15(1):45–66.

[30] Malik P, Bogetti D, Sileri P, et al. Spur cell anemia in alcoholic cirrhosis: cure by orthotopic liver transplantation and recurrence after liver graft failure. Int Surg 2002;87(4):201–4.

[31] Watt K, Uhanova J, Minuk GY. Hepatorenal syndrome: diagnostic accuracy, clinical features, and outcome in a tertiary care center. Am J Gastroenterol 2002;97(8):2046–50.

[32] Cardenas A, Arroyo V. Hepatorenal syndrome. Ann Hepatol 2003;2(1):23–9.

[33] Gines P, Guevara M, Arroyo V, et al. Hepatorenal syndrome. Lancet 2003;362(9398):1819–27.

[34] Sort P, Navasa M, Arroyo V, et al. Effect of intravenous albumin on renal impairment and mortality in patients with cirrhosis and spontaneous bacterial peritonitis. N Engl J Med 1999; 341(6):403–9.

[35] Gong Z, Wezeman FH. Inhibitory effect of alcohol on osteogenic differentiation in human bone marrow-derived mesenchymal stem cells. Alcohol Clin Exp Res 2004;28(3):468–79.

[36] Schnitzler CM, Pieczkowski WM, Fredlund V, et al. Histomorphometric analysis of osteopenia associated with endemic osteoarthritis [Mseleni joint disease]. Bone 1988;9(1):21–7.

[37] Bikle DD, Stesin A, Halloran B, et al. Alcohol-induced bone disease: relationship to age and parathyroid hormone levels. Alcohol Clin Exp Res 1993;17(3):690–5.

[38] Peris P, Pares A, Guanabens N, et al. Reduced spinal and femoral bone mass and deranged bone mineral metabolism in chronic alcoholics. Alcohol Alcohol 1992;27(6):619–25.

[39] American Gastroenterological Association medical position statement. Osteoporosis in hepatic disorders. Gastroenterology 2003;125(3):937–40.

[40] Leslie WD, Bernstein CN, Leboff MS. AGA technical review on osteoporosis in hepatic disorders. Gastroenterology 2003;125(3):941–66.

[41] Fallon MB, Abrams GA. Hepatopulmonary syndrome. Curr Gastroenterol Rep 2000;2(1): 40–5.

[42] Cornely CM, Schade RR, Van Thiel DH, et al. Chronic advanced liver disease and impotence: cause and effect? Hepatology 1984;4(6):1227–30.

[43] Farnsworth WE, Cavanaugh AH, Brown JR, et al. Factors underlying infertility in the alcoholic. Arch Androl 1978;1(2):193–5.

[44] Van Steenbergen W. Alcohol, liver cirrhosis and disorders in sex hormone metabolism. Acta Clin Belg 1993;48(4):269–83.

[45] Van Thiel DH, Gavaler JS, Sanghvi A. Recovery of sexual function in abstinent alcoholic men. Gastroenterology 1983;84(4):677–82.

[46] Zein NN, Abdulkarim AS, Wiesner RH, et al. Prevalence of diabetes mellitus in patients with end-stage liver cirrhosis due to hepatitis C, alcohol, or cholestatic disease. J Hepatol 2000; 32(2):209–17.

[47] Blei AT, Cordoba J. Hepatic encephalopathy. Am J Gastroenterol 2001;96(7):1968–76.

[48] Mullen KD. Newer aspects of hepatic encephalopathy. Indian J Gastroenterol 2003;22(Suppl 2): S17–20.

[49] Mullen KD. Interplay of portal pressure, portal perfusion and hepatic arterial inflow in modulating expression of hepatic encephalopathy in patients with spontaneous or artificially created portosystemic shunts. Indian J Gastroenterol 2003;22(Suppl 2):S25–7.

[50] Siegerstetter V, Rossle M. The role of TIPS for the treatment of portal hypertension: effects and efficacy. Acta Gastroenterol Belg 1997;60(3):233–7.

[51] Bureau C, Garcia-Pagan JC, Otal P, et al. Improved clinical outcome using polytetrafluoro-ethylene-coated stents for TIPS: results of a randomized study. Gastroenterology 2004;126(2): 469–75.

[52] Rossle M, Mullen KD. Long-term patency is expected with covered TIPS stents: this effect may not always be desirable! Hepatology 2004;40(2):495–7.

[53] Morikawa S, Kumada K, Fukui K, et al. Closure of interposition mesocaval shunt in a case of idiopathic portal hypertension. Am J Gastroenterol 1989;84(5):548–51.

[54] Ferenci P, Lockwood A, Mullen K, et al. Hepatic encephalopathy–definition, nomenclature, diagnosis, and quantification: final report of the working party at the 11th World Congresses of Gastroenterology, Vienna, 1998. Hepatology 2002;35(3):716–21.

[55] Arguedas MR, DeLawrence TG, McGuire BM. Influence of hepatic encephalopathy on health-related quality of life in patients with cirrhosis. Dig Dis Sci 2003;48(8):1622–6.

[56] Srivastava A, Mehta R, Rothke SP, et al. Fitness to drive in patients with cirrhosis and portal-systemic shunting: a pilot study evaluating driving performance. J Hepatol 1994;21(6):1023–8.

[57] Wein C, Koch H, Popp B, et al. Minimal hepatic encephalopathy impairs fitness to drive. Hepatology 2004;39(3):739–45.

[58] McCrea M, Cordoba J, Vessey G, et al. Neuropsychological characterization and detection of subclinical hepatic encephalopathy. Arch Neurol 1996;53(8):758–63.

[59] Cordoba J, Lopez-Hellin J, Planas M, et al. Normal protein diet for episodic hepatic encephalopathy: results of a randomized study. J Hepatol 2004;41(1):38–43.

[60] Mullen KD, Dasarathy S. Protein restriction in hepatic encephalopathy: necessary evil or illogical dogma? J Hepatol 2004 Jul;41(1):147–8.

[61] Stickel F, Hoehn B, Schuppan D, et al. Review article: nutritional therapy in alcoholic liver disease. Aliment Pharmacol Ther 2003;18(4):357–73.

[62] Srivastava N, Singh N, Joshi YK. Nutrition in the management of hepatic encephalopathy. Trop Gastroenterol 2003;24(2):59–62.

[63] Zavaglia C, Brivio M, Losacco E, et al. The dietary protein contribution and hepatic encephalopathy in cirrhosis. [Italian] Recenti Prog Med 1992;83(4):218–23.

[64] Pelletier G, Roulot D, Davion T, et al. A randomized controlled trial of ursodeoxycholic acid in patients with alcohol-induced cirrhosis and jaundice. Hepatology 2003;37(4):887–92.

[65] Rambaldi A, Iaquinto G, Gluud C. Anabolic-androgenic steroids for alcoholic liver disease: a Cochrane review. Am J Gastroenterol 2002;97(7):1674–81.

[66] Rambaldi A, Gluud C. Propylthiouracil for alcoholic liver disease. Cochrane Database Syst Rev 2002;2:CD002800.

[67] Cortez-Pinto H, Alexandrino P, Camilo ME, et al. Lack of effect of colchicine in alcoholic cirrhosis: final results of a double blind randomized trial. Eur J Gastroenterol Hepatol 2002; 14(4):377–81.

[68] Rambaldi A, Gluud C. Colchicine for alcoholic and non-alcoholic liver fibrosis and cirrhosis. Cochrane Database Syst Rev 2001;3:CD002148.

[69] Ferenci P, Dragosics B, Dittrich H, et al. Randomized controlled trial of silymarin treatment in patients with cirrhosis of the liver. J Hepatol 1989;9(1):105–13.

[70] Wellington K, Jarvis B. Silymarin: a review of its clinical properties in the management of hepatic disorders. BioDrugs 2001;15(7):465–89.

[71] Pares A, Planas R, Torres M, et al. Effects of silymarin in alcoholic patients with cirrhosis of the liver: results of a controlled, double-blind, randomized and multicenter trial. J Hepatol 1998; 28(4):615–21.

[72] Lieber CS. S-adenosyl-L-methionine and alcoholic liver disease in animal models: implications for early intervention in human beings. Alcohol 2002;27(3):173–7.

[73] Rambaldi A, Gluud C. S-adenosyl-L-methionine for alcoholic liver diseases. Cochrane Database Syst Rev 2001;4:CD002235.

[74] Campillo B, Richardet JP, Scherman E, et al. Evaluation of nutritional practice in hospitalized cirrhotic patients: results of a prospective study. Nutrition 2003;19(6):515–21.

[75] Tessari P. Protein metabolism in liver cirrhosis: from albumin to muscle myofibrils. Curr Opin Clin Nutr Metab Care 2003;6(1):79–85.

[76] Andersen H, Borre M, Jakobsen J, et al. Decreased muscle strength in patients with alcoholic liver cirrhosis in relation to nutritional status, alcohol abstinence, liver function, and neuropathy. Hepatology 1998;27(5):1200–6.

[77] Muller MJ. Malnutrition in cirrhosis. J Hepatol 1995;23(Suppl 1):31–5.

[78] Franco D, Belghiti J, Cortesse A, et al. Nutritional status and immunity in alcoholic cirrhosis (author's transl). Gastroenterol Clin Biol 1981;5(10):839–46.

[79] Mendenhall CL, Anderson S, Weesner RE, et al. Protein-calorie malnutrition associated with alcoholic hepatitis. Veterans Administration Cooperative Study Group on Alcoholic Hepatitis. Am J Med 1984;76(2):211–22.

[80] Kovacs EJ. Influence of alcohol and gender on immune response. National Institute on Alcohol Abuse and Alcoholism. Available at: www.niaaa.nih.gov/publications. Accessed 2002.

[81] Hirsch S, de la Maza MP, Gattas V, et al. Nutritional support in alcoholic cirrhotic patients improves host defenses. J Am Coll Nutr 1999;18(5):434–41.

[82] Aagaard NK, Andersen H, Vilstrup H, et al. Muscle strength, Na,K-pumps, magnesium and potassium in patients with alcoholic liver cirrhosis–relation to spironolactone. J Intern Med 2002;252(1):56–63.

[83] Westphal JF, Brogard JM. Drug administration in chronic liver disease. Drug Saf 1997;17(1): 47–73.

[84] Chalasani N, Said A, Ness R, et al. Screening for hepatocellular carcinoma in patients with cirrhosis in the United States: results of a national survey. Am J Gastroenterol 1999; 94(8):2224–9.

[85] Bruix J, Sherman M, Llovet JM, et al. Clinical management of hepatocellular carcinoma. Conclusions of the Barcelona-2000 EASL conference. European Association for the Study of the Liver. J Hepatol 2001;35(3):421–30.

[86] National Institutes of Health Consensus Development Conference Panel statement. Management of hepatitis C. Hepatology 1997;26(3 Suppl 1):2S–10S.

[87] Starzl TE, Van Thiel D, Tzakis AG, et al. Orthotopic liver transplantation for alcoholic cirrhosis. JAMA 1988;260(17):2542–4.

[88] Tome S, Martinez-Rey C, Gonzalez-Quintela A, et al. Influence of superimposed alcoholic hepatitis on the outcome of liver transplantation for end-stage alcoholic liver disease. J Hepatol 2002;36(6):793–8.

[89] Pageaux GP, Perney P, Larrey D. Liver transplantation for alcoholic liver disease. Addict Biol 2001;6(4):301–8.

[90] Yates WR, Martin M, LaBrecque D, et al. A model to examine the validity of the 6-month abstinence criterion for liver transplantation. Alcohol Clin Exp Res 1998;22(2):513–7.

[91] Jauhar S, Talwalkar JA, Schneekloth T, et al. Analysis of factors that predict alcohol relapse following liver transplantation. Liver Transplant 2004;10(3):408–11.

[92] Tome S, Lucey MR. Timing of liver transplantation in alcoholic cirrhosis. J Hepatol 2003; 39(3):302–7.

[93] Neuberger J, Schulz KH, Day C, et al. Transplantation for alcoholic liver disease. J Hepatol 2002;36(1):130–7.

ELSEVIER
SAUNDERS

Clin Liver Dis 9 (2005) 151–169

Alcohol in Hepatocellular Cancer

Michael D. Voigt, MBChB, M.Med, FCP(SA)

4553E JCP, 200 Hawkins Drive, Iowa City, IA 52245, USA

Hepatocellular cancer accounts for almost half a million cancer deaths a year [1–3], with an escalating incidence in the Western world [4–8]. Alcohol has long been recognized as a major risk factor for cancer of the liver and of other organs including oropharynx, larynx, esophagus, and possibly the breast and colon [9–14]. There is compelling epidemiologic data confirming the increased risk of cancer associated with alcohol consumption, which is supported by animal experiments. Cancer of the liver associated with alcohol usually occurs in the setting of cirrhosis [15]. Alcohol may act as a cocarcinogen, and has strong synergistic effects with other carcinogens including hepatitis B and C, aflatoxin, vinyl chloride, obesity and diabetes mellitus. Acetaldehyde, the main metabolite of alcohol, causes hepatocellular injury, and is an important factor in causing increased oxidant stress, which damages DNA. Alcohol affects nutrition and vitamin metabolism, causing abnormalities of DNA methylation. Abnormalities of DNA methylation, a key pathway of epigenetic gene control, lead to cancer. Other nutritional and metabolic effects, for example on vitamin A metabolism, also play a key role in hepatocarcinogenesis. Alcohol enhances the effects of environmental carcinogens directly and by contributing to nutritional deficiency and impairing immunological tumor surveillance. This review summarizes the epidemiologic evidence for the role of alcohol in hepatocellular cancer, and discusses the mechanisms involved in the promotion of cancer.

This article was supported by the Maahs Family Trust.
E-mail address: Michael-Voigt@Uiowa.edu

Epidemiology of alcohol in cancer

Alcohol is a major cause of cirrhosis and cancer

Alcohol is the most common of the known risk factors for hepatocellular cancer (HCC) in the United States [16], where it outstrips hepatitis C (HCV) as a cause of HCC. Between 1993 and 1995, the age-adjusted risk for HCC due to alcohol was approximately five times greater than that for hepatitis C. It remains approximately 1.8 times more common as a cause for HCC than hepatitis C, despite the recent large increase in HCC due to hepatitis C [16] (Fig. 1). The importance of alcohol in HCC varies geographically, along with the marked geographic variation in the incidence of HCC. In geographic areas with high incidence rates of HCC, such as Africa and Asia, the dominant effect of hepatitis B (HBV), HCV, and aflatoxin dilute the effects of alcohol in causing HCC. In these areas, 40% to 50% of cancers occur in noncirrhotic livers [17]. In northern Europe and the United States, approximately 80% to 90% percent of hepatocellular cancers develop in cirrhotic livers. In these areas, cirrhosis is thus the primary predisposing factor for developing hepatocellular cancer. The importance of alcohol as a cause of cirrhosis in the United States and Europe is well established. Best available estimates are that alcoholic liver disease accounts for 40% of deaths from cirrhosis, and 28% of deaths attributed to liver disease in the United States [18]. This is supported by transplantation data for end-stage liver disease, where alcoholic cirrhosis accounts for approximately 17% to 22% of transplants done in the United States and Europe, despite stricter selection than other conditions [19,20]. This is the second leading indication for transplantation, after hepatitis C [19,20].

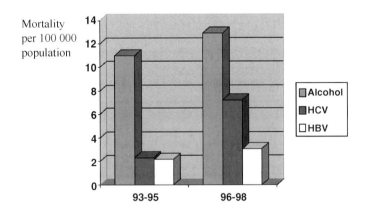

Fig. 1. The age-adjusted hospitalization rate per 100,000 population for alcohol, HCV, and HBV-induced hepatocellular cancer, in the years 1993 to 1995, and 1996 to 1998. (*From* El Serag HB, Mason AC. Risk factors for the rising rates of primary liver cancer in the Uniterd States. Arch Intern Med 2000;150:3227–30; with permission.)

Table 1
Risk factors for hepatocellular cancer

Risk factor	Europe	Japan	Africa/Asia
HBV	<15	20	60
HCV	60	50	<10
Alcohol	<15	<20	20

Data from Bosch F, Ribes J, Borras J. Epidemiology of primary liver cancer. Semin Liver Dis 1999; 19:271–85.

In all cirrhotic patients, the annual risk of developing HCC is 2% to 6% (summarized by Collier and Sherman [21]). The risk of cancer developing in cirrhosis increases with age, and among other factors, more advanced disease [22–24]. The risk attributable to alcohol is compared with HBV and HCV in different geographic regions, and is summarized in Table 1 [24a].

There is a strong association between the risk of hepatocellular cancer and alcohol consumption [25]. Epidemiologic studies have shown a strong dose–response relationship between alcohol intake and risk of cancer [26,27]. Many other studies have shown an increased risk with an arbitrarily chosen level of high alcohol intake [28–34]. The risk is similar for men and women. Interestingly, the risk was found to be higher for former drinkers than those who continued to drink. This increased risk remained for at least 10 years after quitting [26]. This "reverse cause–effect" relationship, where risk remains despite quitting alcohol use, may be explained by the fact that subjects stop drinking when they develop early symptoms or signs of liver disease. As the liver disease remains after quitting alcohol, the risk of cancer remains. In addition, a proportion of subjects who continue to drink will die from complications of alcohol use, and not live long enough for cancer to manifest. This reverse cause–effect relationship to quitting alcohol is not unique to liver cancer, but has also been shown for other upper aero-digestive tract cancers (esophagus, larynx, and pharynx) [35,36]. As with liver cancer, the peak risk for these cancers occurs shortly after stopping alcohol use, and there is no clear decline up to 10 years after stopping [35,36].

Long-term intake of small amounts of alcohol does not increase the risk of cancer [26,27,37]. However, larger "toxic" amounts, taken over a shorter period, do increase the risk. These findings also apply in upper digestive tract cancer [35,36,38,39].

The discussion of alcohol as a risk factor for hepatocellular cancer would not be complete without pointing out that several large population-based studies have shown results that contradict the role of alcohol in causing cancer.

Kuper et al [40] showed that in 1556 patients with coexistent chronic viral hepatitis B or C and alcoholism without cirrhosis, no additional risk was attributable to alcohol beyond that linked to hepatitis alone.

Similarly, in a large prospective study of 90,000 patients in Haimen City, China, alcohol consumption was not significantly associated with hepatocellular cancer. Indeed, analysis of 35,171 heavy drinkers, including 9348 who drank >100 g of alcohol on the days they drank, there was a slight protective effect of moderate alcohol use (relative risk 0.83, confidence interval [CI] 0.72–0.95) [41]. Sun et al [42], in a population study of 12,008 subjects, also showed that alcohol use did not act as a significant risk factor alone, in causing HCC (relative ratio [RR] 1.5 CI 1.0–2.3], although the combination of alcohol and HCV showed an increased risk compared with HCV alone.

Confounding factors that may explain these discrepant findings include the potential bias of questionnaires for alcohol recall. The apparent protective effect of alcohol in hospital-based studies could be explained by early death caused by ongoing alcohol use, before cancer can manifest, in patients admitted to the hospital with alcoholic hepatitis. Population-based studies are also prone to mislabeling subjects with other forms of cirrhosis, as having alcoholic cirrhosis, if they drink.

Alcohol acts synergistically with other carcinogens

There is a strong synergistic effect of alcohol use with other carcinogens and cocarcinogens [26].

Alcohol and smoking

Several studies suggest that there is an interactive effect of heavy smoking and heavy drinking on the development of HCC [43]. Kuper showed a super multiplicative effect of heavy smoking and heavy drinking in the development of HCC (odds ratio [OR] for both exposures = 9.6, versus OR = 1.9 for alcohol alone) [44]. Similarly, Mukaiya showed the relative risk for combination smoking and drinking to be 17.9 [43]. The synergistic effect of alcohol was shown in another way by Ohnishi et al [45]. They found that as the number of risk factors (including smoking, alcohol HBV, and HCV) for HCC increased, the latency period for developing HCC got progressively shorter [45].

Although combined alcohol use and smoking are clearly synergistic in caus-ing cancer, data on the risk of HCC with smoking alone (in the absence of heavy alcohol use) are contradictory, with some studies showing a dose–response rela-tionship [46,47] and others showing no significant association [48,49]. Taking these observations together, it is postulated that carcinogenic compounds in cigarette smoke have an increased effect in the presence of heavy alcohol use, as they exert their carcinogenicity in the context of liver injury, which causes cellular proliferation from injury repair, which predisposes the liver to developing cancer. In addition, the liver plays an important role in metabolizing carcinogens absorbed from tobacco use [50]. CYP2E1 induction by alcohol may alter and enhance the carcinogenic potential of agents in tobacco [44].

Alcohol and hepatitis B and hepatitis C

Alcohol use substantially increases the risk that HCC will develop in subjects with HBV or HCV. This has been shown in case–control studies where the RR of

HCC for the combination of alcohol use HBV or HCV is substantially greater than the RR of viral hepatitis alone [51–53]. HBV infection is more common in alcoholics than nonalcoholics, and patients with worse liver disease have a higher the prevalence of HBV markers [54]. This is also true for hepatitis C [54–59].

HCC occurs 10 years earlier in HBV-positive subjects who drink than in HBV-positive subjects who do not drink [60]. HCV is more common in alcoholic than nonalcoholic patients, and the prevalence of HCV is the greatest in alcoholic patients with the most advanced liver disease [58]. Alcoholic patients with HCV also have worse disease than those without HCV, as shown by higher alanine amino transferase (ALT) values and higher disease activity on liver histology [61]. HCV RNA levels and liver disease severity are higher in alcohol users than nondrinkers [57,62].

The synergistic effect of viral hepatitis and alcohol use in causing HCC, may thus at least be partly explained by the alcohol and hepatitis viruses acting in concert to make the liver disease worse, which hastens the development of cirrhosis and increases its severity. The more advanced the cirrhosis, the greater the risk of cancer. Additionally, the use of alcohol may enhance the carcinogenic potential of hepatitis viruses.

Alcohol and diabetes mellitus

Patients with severe obesity have a nearly fivefold increased risk of developing liver cancer [63], which may be due to an increased risk of cirrhosis from NASH or because of the effects of high insulin levels and insulin-like growth factors stimulating hepatocyte proliferation [64]. Both diabetes and alcohol on their own increase the risk of HCC. However, when diabetes and heavy alcohol use occur together, the risk of cancer is increased substantially more than the additive risk for each condition [34,51,65].

The mechanisms of the strong synergy between diabetes and alcohol use in causing cancer are unknown. Complications of diabetes mellitus may be caused by increased oxidative stress [66–68], which may be mediated in part by altered iron metabolism in diabetics [69]. The effect of alcohol in promoting oxidative stress, and the effects of oxidative stress in leading to cancer, are described below. Other mediators are likely to be of importance.

Alcohol and vinyl chloride

Like alcohol, vinyl chloride exposure on its own increases the risk of HCC about 70% to 300% [70–73]. Mastrangelo et al. [72] showed that for every 1000 ppm×years of vinyl chloride cumulative exposure, the risk of HCC increased by 71%. The combined effect of vinyl chloride exposure above 2500 ppm × years and alcohol intake above 60 g/d resulted in a massive increase in the OR to 409 (95% CI, 19.6–8553) for HCC. This shows a clear synergistic rather than additive effect, suggesting the two agents interact biologically to increase the risk of HCC. The biologic interaction is postulated to include several mechanisms. First, alcohol induces cytochrome 2E1 (CYP2E1) [74], which is primarily responsible for converting vinyl chloride to chloroethylene oxide and chloracetaldehyde. These toxic metabolites of vinyl chloride have been shown to be mutagenic in multiple models. Alcohol reduces glutathione levels in the liver, and hence, it impairs the protective arm of the vinyl chloride metabolism by reducing the ability to detoxify vinyl chloride metabolites [75,76]. CYP2E1 upregulation also increases catabolism of retinoic acid (RA), which enhances cellular proliferation by upregulation of the AP-1 (c-jun and c-fos) transcriptional complex [77]. This increased cellular proliferation occurs in the environment of increased reactive oxygen species caused by alcohol metabolism to acetaldehyde. The reactive oxygen species enhance DNA damage and impair DNA adduct removal [78]. In addition, alcohol and vinyl chloride both promote liver fibrosis, and ultimately cirrhosis hyperadditively [72,79].

Alcohol and aflatoxin

Aflatoxin B1 (AFB1) is a major hepatocarcinogen, which acts in part by causing mutations of codon 249, a mutational hotspot of the p53 tumor suppressor gene [80,81]. Aflatoxin is metabolized by CYP2E1, which is induced by alcohol. Thus, alcohol use increases the genotoxic effect of AFB1. Epidemiologic evidence suggests that use of as little as 24 g/d of ethanol increases the risk of developing HCC induced AFB1 by 35-fold [82].

Mechanisms of alcohol-induced hepatocellular cancer

Heavy alcohol use induces HCC predominantly by causing cirrhosis. Several epidemiologic studies suggest that liver cirrhosis is the most important intermediate step in producing HCC. However, there may be a small additional risk of cancer developing due to carcinogenic or cocarcinogenic effects of alcohol. This (co-)carcinogenic effect of alcohol, however, appears to be less for HCC than for cancers of the oropharynx, esophagus, and larynx [10,83].

In a large population-based study from Sweden of 186,395 patients, alcoholic patients without cirrhosis had a 2.4-fold risk of developing hepatocellular cancer, compared with the general population. The risk was many times greater (22.4) in alcohol users if cirrhosis was present. The increased cancer risk with alcohol use in the absence of cirrhosis suggests that alcohol has a direct carcinogenic effects. However, the authors speculated that preclinical cirrhosis may have been present in those developing cancer [40]. In this study, cirrhosis alone, in the absence of viral hepatitis and alcoholism, was associated with a 40-fold relative risk for HCC [40].

Additional data confirming the prime importance of cirrhosis as an intermediate condition that is generally required for cancer to develop comes from prospective cohort studies of cirrhotics. In 463 prospectively followed cirrhotics, including 59% with cirrhosis due to alcohol, multivariate analysis failed to show alcohol as an additional risk factor for HCC. The 4-year cumulative risk of cancer in the alcoholic cirrhotics was 15.3%, which was not significantly different from 11.9% in the nondrinking cirrhotics [24]. This also implies that alcohol is at least as carcinogenic as the nonalcohol causes of cirrhosis (such as HBV and HCV), which lead to cancer. Retrospective studies using multivariate analysis have also failed to show an increased risk associated with alcohol once cirrhosis is present [84]. Some case–control studies have shown that alcohol consumption may be negatively associated with cancer risk [85]. Ongoing alcohol use in cirrhotics, resulting in death before cancer could manifest, likely accounts for these discrepant findings. This confounding effect could also mask the effects of alcohol in population-based studies.

Acetaldehyde as a carcinogen

Chronic ethanol use causes continual hepatocyte destruction through the metabolic effects resulting from alcohol metabolism [86]. Both altered redox state and acetaldehyde production may be important. Acetaldehyde, the product of ethanol metabolism by alcohol dehydrogenase (ADH) is an important carcinogen in humans and animals [87], and has also been shown to be primarily responsible for alcohol-induced hepatocyte injury [88]. Acetaldehyde binds to cellular proteins and DNA. It impairs DNA repair, and affects sister chromatid exchange, which in part accounts for its mutagenic, carcinogenic, and teratogenic effects [89–92]. It also causes cellular injury, which leads to cellular proliferation and regeneration, and ultimately to cirrhosis [88–92].

The toxic effects of acetaldehyde depend on the total hepatocyte exposure (dose) to acetaldehyde. This depends on how quickly acetaldehyde is formed from ethanol, by the action of ADH, and how quickly it metabolized to nontoxic acetate, by aldehyde dehydrogenase (ALDH). Both alcohol and acetaldehyde dehydrogenase enzymes are polymorphic. Alleles ADH2*2 and ADH3*1, which encode for high-capacity enzymes, produce acetaldehyde more rapidly, increase exposure to acetaldehyde, and have been shown to increase risk of alcoholic liver disease [93]. Similarly, polymorphisms of acetaldehyde dehydrogenase, which are relatively less active (ALDH2*2), and hence metabolize acetaldehyde slowly, tend to increase acetaldehyde exposure. Several studies have shown an increased risk of cancer in Japanese drinkers with ALDH2 [30,94,95]. Munaka showed that in drinkers with either ALDH2*2 or 2*1, the risk of cancer was increased (OR = 2.53, 95% CI 1.21–5.31) [30]. Ohhira found ALDH 2*1 in all patients with alcoholic cirrhosis who developed cancer [94]. Not all studies have shown this association [96].

Cytochrome P450 2E1 and alcohol in hepatocellular cancer

Alcohol use may contribute to hepatocarcinogenesis by inducing CYP2E1. The increased activity of CYP2E1 has been shown to enhance conversion of procarcinogens to carcinogens. Examples include dimethylnitrosamines, benzene, and aniline, aflatoxin B1 (AFB1), vinyl chloride, and dimethylhydrazine [97–99]. The c2 genetic polymorphism of CYP2E1 confers higher activity, hence, an enhanced potential to activate procarcinogens. The presence of the c2 allele is associated with a four- to sixfold increased risk of HCC in alcoholic patients [30,100,101], although controversy exists [102]. Alcohol use not only enhances CYP2E1 activity, but also may increase carcinogen and procarcinogen absorption, and alcohol use is commonly associated with cigarette smoking, which is a rich source of carcinogens.

If DNA adducts from the metabolites of procarcinogens are not repaired, they may lead to mutations when cell division occurs. Accumulation of these mutations may lead to cancer through interference with genomic integrity [103].

Alcohol and oxidative stress in hepatocarcinogenesis

Another important mechanism of alcohol induction of cancer is in the production of oxidative stress. Alcohol metabolism by CYP2E1 plays an important role in causing oxidant stress, which is enhanced by induction of CYP2E1 by alcohol. The mechanism by which CYP2E1 induces oxidant stress has recently been reviewed [104,105].

Heavy alcohol use also causes generation of reactive oxygen and reactive nitrogen species by parenchymal cells in response to cytokine-induced stress signals and by activation of Kupffer cells and infiltrating inflammatory cells [106,107].

Alcohol also aggravates oxidant stress caused by viral hepatitis [108], which may explain the synergistic carcinogenetic effect between alcohol abuse and viral hepatitis. Chronic alcohol abuse, and the frequent accompanying malnutrition, may deplete antioxidant defenses (see below).

Oxidant stress occurs when excessive production of reactive oxygen and nitrogen species overwhelms the antioxidant defense system's ability to clear the reactive molecules. The antioxidant defense system includes glutathione, α-tocopherol, superoxide dismutase, catalase, and glutathione peroxidase. Reactive oxygen and nitrogen species are highly reactive radicals that cause lipid peroxidation of poly-unsaturated fatty acids, and produce reactive aldehydes such as malondialdehyde and trans-4-hydroxy-2-nonenal (HNE) [109]. These electrophilic by-products of lipid peroxidation in turn react with DNA bases and form exocyclic DNA adducts (examples include 1,N6-ethenodeoxyadenosine and 3,N4-ethenodeoxycytidine, trans-4-hydroxy-2-nonenal [4-HNE]) [110]. These adducts may lead to mutation and disruption of genomic integrity, including inactivation of tumor suppressor genes, ultimately initiating cancer. For example, 4-HNE–DNA adducts have been shown to preferentially bind the third base of codon 249, a mutational hotspot in the p53 gene. This major electrophilic product of lipid peroxidation may be an important etiologic agent for hepatocellular cancer by causing mutations that suppress the p53 gene [111].

Alcohol folate, B6, B12, metabolism, and DNA methylation in hepatocellular cancer

Heavy alcohol use may lead to nutritional deficiency of vitamins and trace elements through intake of "empty calories", malabsorption, and destruction of vitamins by alcohol. Oxidative stress caused by heavy alcohol use depletes antioxidants [15,112].

Chronic alcohol interacts with intake, absorption, and subsequent metabolism of vitamins involved in hepatic transmethylation reactions. The most important of these are folate, vitamin B12, and pyridoxal-5'-phosphate (vitamin B6) [113–119]. Deficiency of these agents caused by heavy alcohol use, results in impaired hepatic methyl group synthesis and transfer [113–119], which may affect DNA methylation, and hence, epigenetic control of genes involved in hepatocarcinogenesis.

Heavy alcohol use leads to diminished folate stores through a variety of mechanisms.

1. Alcohol impairs translation and activity of intestinal reduced folate carrier, which impairs intestinal folate absorption [113–119].
2. Alcohol directly inhibits hepatic folate uptake [120].
3. Alcohol reduces renal folate conservation [121], leading to increased folate excretion, even in the face of folate deficiency.

This all results in impaired hepatic methyl group synthesis and transfer, which results in reduced levels of the most important antioxidants, hepatic methionine, S-adenosylmethionine (SAM) [122], and glutathione. As a consequence, markers for DNA and lipid oxidation are increased [120]. Chronic alcohol use also interferes with intake, absorption and metabolism of vitamin B6, which further impairs hepatic methyl group synthesis and transfer. Alcohol consumption also impairs vitamin B12 metabolism [123]. Nutritional deficiency and metabolic impairment of any one of folate B6 and B12 vitamins, as a consequence of chronic alcohol intake, has been shown in many studies [124,125].

Through the effects on folate B6 and B12 metabolism, alcohol intake has a marked effect on hepatic methylation capacity, resulting in reduced levels of SAM, an important methyl group donor, which results in increased levels of S-adenosylhomocysteine (SAH). The SAM/SAH ratio may be decreased 2.5-fold by alcohol use [126,127].

The effect of alcohol on folate and B6, especially, is clinically important. Deficiency in alcoholics results in elevation in plasma homocysteine levels, which has been shown to be an excellent marker for severe alcohol dependence [128]. Elevated homocysteine is a marker for impaired methylation and trans-sulfuration pathways. In methylation, homocysteine acquires a methyl group from N-5-methyltetrahydrofolate in a vitamin B12-dependent reaction. In the trans-sulfuration pathway, homocysteine condenses with serine to form cystathionine in an irreversible reaction catalyzed by the pyridoxal-5'-phosphate-containing enzyme, cystathionine-beta-synthase [124]. Ethanol also reduces the activity of methionine synthetase, which remethylates homocysteine to methionine [129,130]. Chronic alcohol consumption also reduces glutathione levels, which is synthesized from homocysteine via trans-sulfuration in the liver [130,131]. In addition, alcohol use has also been shown to inhibit activity of DNA methylase, which transfers methyl groups to DNA [132,133].

The consequences of both the altered methylation pathways and the reduced hepatic methionine, glutathione, and SAM has multiple important consequences for hepatocarcinogenesis. Folate and methionine deficiency reliably induces hepatocellular cancer in animal models. The carcinomas correlate with altered DNA methylation in the liver, where cancer develops, but not other tissues, where cancer does not develop. Alterations in DNA methylation occurs early in the preneoplastic stages of carcinogenesis [134].

Altered DNA methylation is an important epigenetic mechanism that affects transcriptional regulation of genes important in hepatocellular cancer. Promoter hypermethylation silences cyclooxygenase-2 and regulates growth in HCC [135]. Hypermethylation of the promotor for hepatocyte growth factor activator inhibitor 2/placental bikunin (HAI-2/PB) gene is associated with the reduced expression of the HAI-2/PB gene in HCC tumors [136]. Suppressor of cytokine signaling-1 (SOCS-1), a tumor suppressor gene, is a negative regulator of Janus kinase and signal transducer and activation of transcription pathways. Aberrant methylation of SOCS-1 methylation may be a key event for HCC transformation of cirrhotic nodules [137]. Multiple other genes important in hepatocellular carcinogenesis, have been shown to have abnormal hyper- or hypomethylation profiles [137–148]. Thus, dietary deficiency of folate, B12, and B6, with resultant altered methionine and methyl-transferase pathways, play a key role in alcohol-related carcinogenesis by altering DNA methylation.

The importance of altered DNA methylation and its interactions with alcohol use is further influenced by polymorphism of key enzymes of folate metabolism that increase the risk of cancer in alcoholics. Methylenetetrahydrofolate reductase (MTHFR), is a key enzyme in folate metabolism, and has a critical role in providing methyl groups for DNA methylation and in the production of deoxy thymidine monophosphate for DNA synthesis. The MTHFR gene has genetic polymorphisms that cause reduced enzyme activity. Impaired folate metabolism by these genetic variants of MTHFR is associated with changes in DNA (including promotor) methylation patterns. One of the less active polymorphisms (CC genotype) of this enzyme, is associated with a >200% increase in the risk of HCC in alcoholics [149]. The importance of genetic polymorphisms of this particular enzyme is confirmed by the fact that is also associated with a markedly increased risk of many other cancers [150–153].

Retinoids and alcohol

Deficiency or abnormal metabolism of vitamin A, and its major metabolite retinoic acid (RA), alters the growth and differentiation of different tumor cell lines in vitro and suppress tumor development in animal models [154]. Vitamin A metabolites bind two classes of nuclear receptors, RA receptors, and retinoid X receptors, members of the steroid/thyroid hormone receptor family. Retinoid treatment may inhibit tumor growth by suppressing cell proliferation, promoting cellular differentiation, and inducing apoptotic cell death [155,156]. These effects are in part mediated by a subgroup of the transforming growth factor-beta superfamily, the bone morphogenetic proteins that act on serine and threonine kinase receptors [157]. Multiple studies have demonstrated an association between vitamin A deficiency and the risk of developing cancer, and this has led to the wide use of vitamin A in the prevention and treatment of cancer [154–156]. The biochemistry and mechanisms of vitamin A metabolites in cancer prevention and treatment has reently been extensively reviewed [158–162].

Alcohol use causes vitamin A deficiency and affects its metabolism. Alcoholics have reduced serum and hepatic vitamin A and beta-carotene concentrations [130,163,164]. Chronic alcohol consumption affects several aspects of vitamin A metabolism, including retinol absorption, enhanced degradation in the liver, and increased mobilization of retinol from the liver to other organs [164,165]. RA is synthesized from retinol via various enzymatic steps involving microsomal and cytosolic ADH and ALDH. Alcohol use directly affects its metabolism [164,165]. Ethanol use also results in decreased hepatic concentrations of the metabolically active precursors of RA, namely retinol and retinyl esters, and alcohol competitively inhibits retinol oxidation, which impairs RA biosynthesis [77,166]. Alcohol induction of CYP2E1 further increases metabolism of RA into inactive polar metabolites [167]. These changes are associated with up to eightfold overexpression of the AP-1 (c-jun, c-fos), which causes hyperproliferation of hepatocytes [168]. Normal activity of both AP-1 and hepatocyte hyperproliferation is restored with vitamin A supplementation [168].

Thus, vitamin A metabolites, which play a vital role in the control of cellular proliferation and differentiation, are profoundly affected by chronic alcohol use, and may substantially contribute to hepatocarcinogenesis in alcoholics.

Alcohol and immune surveillance

Hepatocellular cancers must evade immune surveillance to be able to expand. There is a complex interaction between cancer cells, their microenvironment, and the immune system. Cells of both innate and adaptive immune systems are relevant in tumor attack. Hepatocellular cancer cells have developed a variety of mechanisms to evade tumor surveillance, including altered Fas ligand expression [169] and altered major histocompatibility complex (MHC) molecule expression [170]. In addition, secretion of mucins and other products may create an immune privileged site [171], while low-level exposure of dendritic cells to apoptotic products of hepatocellular cancer cells may promote tolerance. Immune surveillance may also select cells resistant to immune attack. Tumor evasion of immune surveillance is complex, and has recently been extensively reviewed [171–175].

Both acute (binge drinking) [176,177] and chronic alcohol use affect immunity. Chronic alcohol use impairs both innate and adaptive immunity (for a recent review, see Cook [176]). Several studies have shown an increased risk of cancer metastasis and progression associated with loss of immune surveillance from chronic alcohol use in animal models [178,179] and in human studies [180].

Summary

Alcohol is the most common known cause of cancer in the United States and Europe. It largely mediates this by causing cirrhosis. Alcohol acts synergistically with a variety of other agents that increase the risk of HCC, partly by enhancing and hastening the damage caused to the liver, and partly through its unique perturbation several metabolic pathways, which leads ultimately to DNA damage and impaired control of gene expression. The most important known factors are altered oxidant stress, enhanced absorption and conversion of (pro)-carcinogens, effects on DNA methylation, altered retinoid metabolism, and impaired immune surveillance. Unquestionably, other pathways will be demonstrated in the future. The knowledge of the relevant pathogenetic mechanisms may lead to methods to reduce the risk of HCC developing in alcoholic cirrhotics, as many of the pathways may be susceptible interventions, including simple supplementation of vitamins, and provision of additional antioxidants.

References

[1] Parkin DM. Global cancer statistics in the year 2000. Lancet Oncol 2001;2:533–43.

[2] Parkin DM, Bray F, Ferlay J, et al. Estimating the world cancer burden: Globocan 2000. Int J Cancer 2001;94:153–6.

[3] Shibuya K, Mathers CD, Boschi-Pinto C, et al. Global and regional estimates of cancer mortality and incidence by site: II. Results for the global burden of disease 2000. BMC Cancer 2002;2:37.

[4] Garcia-Torres ML, Zaragoza A, Giner R, et al. Incidence and epidemiological factors of hepatocellular carcinoma in Valencia during the year 2000. Rev Esp Enferm Dig 2003;95: 385–8.

[5] Ikai I, Itai Y, Okita K, et al. Report of the 15th follow-up survey of primary liver cancer. Hepatol Res 2004;28:21–9.

[6] Jemal A, Thomas A, Murray T, et al. Cancer statistics, 2002. CA Cancer J Clin 2002;52:23–47.

[7] Shibuya K, Mathers CD, Boschi-Pinto C, et al. Global and regional estimates of cancer mortality and incidence by site: II. Results for the global burden of disease 2000. BMC Cancer 2002;2:37.

[8] Srivatanakul P, Sriplung H, Deerasamee S. Epidemiology of liver cancer: an overview. Asian Pac J Cancer Prev 2004;5:118–25.

[9] Bagnardi V, Blangiardo M, La Vecchia C, et al. Alcohol consumption and the risk of cancer: a meta-analysis. Alcohol Res Health 2001;25:263–70.

[10] Longnecker MP. Alcohol consumption and risk of cancer in humans: an overview. Alcohol 1995;12:87–96.

[11] Poschl G, Seitz HK. Alcohol and cancer. Alcohol Alcohol 2004;39:155–65.

[12] Poschl G, Stickel F, Wang XD, et al. Alcohol and cancer: genetic and nutritional aspects. Proc Nutr Soc 2004;63:65–71.

[13] Rogers AE, Conner MW. Alcohol and cancer. Adv Exp Med Biol 1986;206:473–95.

[14] Seitz HK, Poschl G, Simanowski UA. Alcohol and cancer. Recent Dev Alcohol 1998;14: 67–95.

[15] Stickel F, Schuppan D, Hahn EG, et al. Cocarcinogenic effects of alcohol in hepatocarcinogenesis. Gut 2002;51:132–9.

[16] El Serag HB, Mason AC. Risk factors for the rising rates of primary liver cancer in the United States. Arch Intern Med 2000;160:3227–30.

[17] Kew MC. Hepatocellular cancer. A century of progress. Clin Liver Dis 2000;4:257–68.

[18] Kim WR, Brown Jr RS, Terrault NA, et al. Burden of liver disease in the United States: summary of a workshop. Hepatology 2002;36:227–42.

[19] Hartley P, Petruckevitch A, Reeves B, et al. The National Liver Transplantation audit: an overview of patients presenting for liver transplantation from 1994 to 1998. On behalf of the Steering Group of the UK Liver Transplantation Audit. Br J Surg 2001;88:52–8.

[20] Jaurrieta E, Casais L, Figueras J, et al. [Analysis of 500 liver transplantations at Bellvitge Hospital, Spain.] Med Clin (Barc) 2000;115:521–9.

[21] Collier J, Sherman M. Screening for hepatocellular carcinoma. Hepatology 1998;27:273–8.

[22] Colombo M, De Franchis R, Del Ninno E, et al. Hepatocellular carcinoma in Italian patients with cirrhosis. N Engl J Med 1991;325:675–80.

[23] Donato MF, Arosio E, Del Ninno E, et al. High rates of hepatocellular carcinoma in cirrhotic patients with high liver cell proliferative activity. Hepatology 2001;34:523–8.

[24] Velazquez RF, Rodriguez M, Navascues CA, et al. Prospective analysis of risk factors for hepatocellular carcinoma in patients with liver cirrhosis. Hepatology 2003;37:520–7.

[24a] Bosch F, Ribes J, Borras J. Epidemiology of primary liver cancer. Semin Liver Dis 1999; 19:271–85.

[25] Prior P. Long-term cancer risk in alcoholism. Alcohol Alcohol 1988;23:163–71.

[26] Donato F, Tagger A, Gelatti U, et al. Alcohol and hepatocellular carcinoma: the effect of lifetime intake and hepatitis virus infections in men and women. Am J Epidemiol 2002; 155:323–31.

[27] Mayans MV, Calvet X, Bruix J, et al. Risk factors for hepatocellular carcinoma in Catalonia, Spain. Int J Cancer 1990;46:378–81.

[28] Chiesa R, Donato F, Tagger A, et al. Etiology of hepatocellular carcinoma in Italian patients with and without cirrhosis. Cancer Epidemiol Biomarkers Prev 2000;9:213–6.

[29] Mohamed AE, Kew MC, Groeneveld HT. Alcohol consumption as a risk factor for hepatocellular carcinoma in urban southern African blacks. Int J Cancer 1992;51:537–41.

[30] Munaka M, Kohshi K, Kawamoto T, et al. Genetic polymorphisms of tobacco- and alcohol-related metabolizing enzymes and the risk of hepatocellular carcinoma. J Cancer Res Clin Oncol 2003;129:355–60.

[31] Tanaka K, Hirohata T, Takeshita S. Blood transfusion, alcohol consumption, and cigarette smoking in causation of hepatocellular carcinoma: a case–control study in Fukuoka, Japan. Jpn J Cancer Res 1988;79:1075–82.

[32] Tsukuma H, Hiyama T, Oshima A, et al. A case–control study of hepatocellular carcinoma in Osaka, Japan. Int J Cancer 1990;45:231–6.

[33] Yang HI, Lu SN, Liaw YF, et al. Hepatitis B e antigen and the risk of hepatocellular carcinoma. N Engl J Med 2002;347:168–74.

[34] Yu MC, Tong MJ, Govindarajan S, et al. Nonviral risk factors for hepatocellular carcinoma in a low-risk population, the non-Asians of Los Angeles County, California. J Natl Cancer Inst 1991;83:1820–6.

[35] Franceschi S, Levi F, Dal Maso L, et al. Cessation of alcohol drinking and risk of cancer of the oral cavity and pharynx. Int J Cancer 2000;85:787–90.

[36] Launoy G, Milan CH, Faivre J, et al. Alcohol, tobacco and oesophageal cancer: effects of the duration of consumption, mean intake and current and former consumption. Br J Cancer 1997;75:1389–96.

[37] Corrao G, Arico S, Lepore R, et al. Amount and duration of alcohol intake as risk factors of symptomatic liver cirrhosis: a case–control study. J Clin Epidemiol 1993;46:601–7.

[38] Castellsague X, Munoz N, De Stefani E, et al. Independent and joint effects of tobacco smoking and alcohol drinking on the risk of esophageal cancer in men and women. Int J Cancer 1999;82:657–64.

[39] Zambon P, Talamini R, La Vecchia C, et al. Smoking, type of alcoholic beverage and squamous-cell oesophageal cancer in northern Italy. Int J Cancer 2000;86:144–9.

[40] Kuper H, Ye W, Broome U, et al. The risk of liver and bile duct cancer in patients with chronic viral hepatitis, alcoholism, or cirrhosis. Hepatology 2001;34:714–8.

[41] Evans AA, Chen G, Ross EA, et al. Eight-year follow-up of the 90,000-person Haimen City cohort: I. Hepatocellular carcinoma mortality, risk factors, and gender differences. Cancer Epidemiol Biomarkers Prev 2002;11:369–76.

[42] Sun CA, Wu DM, Lin CC, et al. Incidence and cofactors of hepatitis C virus-related hepatocellular carcinoma: a prospective study of 12,008 men in Taiwan. Am J Epidemiol 2003; 157:674–82.

[43] Mukaiya M, Nishi M, Miyake H, et al. Chronic liver diseases for the risk of hepatocellular carcinoma: a case–control study in Japan. Etiologic association of alcohol consumption, cigarette smoking and the development of chronic liver diseases. Hepatogastroenterology 1998; 45:2328–32.

[44] Kuper H, Tzonou A, Kaklamani E, et al. Tobacco smoking, alcohol consumption and their interaction in the causation of hepatocellular carcinoma. Int J Cancer 2000;85:498–502.

[45] Ohnishi K, Terabayashi H, Unuma T, et al. Effects of habitual alcohol intake and cigarette smoking on the development of hepatocellular carcinoma. Alcohol Clin Exp Res 1987; 11:45–8.

[46] Tanaka K, Hirohata T, Takeshita S, et al. Hepatitis B virus, cigarette smoking and alcohol consumption in the development of hepatocellular carcinoma: a case–control study in Fukuoka, Japan. Int J Cancer 1992;51:509–14.

[47] Trichopoulos D, Day NE, Kaklamani E, et al. Hepatitis B virus, tobacco smoking and ethanol consumption in the etiology of hepatocellular carcinoma. Int J Cancer 1987;39:45–9.

[48] Hadziyannis S, Tabor E, Kaklamani E, et al. A case–control study of hepatitis B and C virus infections in the etiology of hepatocellular carcinoma. Int J Cancer 1995;60:627–31.

[49] La Vecchia C, Negri E, Decarli A, et al. Risk factors for hepatocellular carcinoma in northern Italy. Int J Cancer 1988;42:872–6.

[50] Staretz ME, Murphy SE, Patten CJ, et al. Comparative metabolism of the tobacco-related carcinogens benzo[a]pyrene, 4-(methylnitrosamino)-1-(3-pyridyl)-1-butanone, 4-(methylnitrosamino)-1-(3-pyridyl)-1-butanol, and N'- nitrosonornicotine in human hepatic microsomes. Drug Metab Dispos 1997;25:154–62.

[51] Hassan MM, Hwang LY, Hatten CJ, et al. Risk factors for hepatocellular carcinoma: synergism of alcohol with viral hepatitis and diabetes mellitus. Hepatology 2002;36:1206–13.

[52] Popper H, Shafritz DA, Hoofnagle JH. Relation of the hepatitis B virus carrier state to hepatocellular carcinoma. Hepatology 1987;7:764–72.

[53] Rosman AS. Viral hepatitis and alcoholism. Alcohol Health Res 1992;16:48–56.

[54] Mendenhall CL, Seeff L, Diehl AM, et al. Antibodies to hepatitis B virus and hepatitis C virus in alcoholic hepatitis and cirrhosis: their prevalence and clinical relevance. The VA Cooperative Study Group (No. 119). Hepatology 1991;14:581–9.

[55] Nalpas B, Thiers V, Pol S, et al. HCV infection in alcoholics. Gastroenterol Jpn 1993; 28(Suppl 5):88–90.

[56] Nishiguchi S, Kuroki T, Yabusako T, et al. Detection of hepatitis C virus antibodies and hepatitis C virus RNA in patients with alcoholic liver disease. Hepatology 1991;14:985–9.

[57] Oshita M, Hayashi N, Kasahara A, et al. Increased serum hepatitis C virus RNA levels among alcoholic patients with chronic hepatitis C. Hepatology 1994;20:1115–20.

[58] Pares A, Barrera JM, Caballeria J, et al. Hepatitis C virus antibodies in chronic alcoholic patients: association with severity of liver injury. Hepatology 1990;12:1295–9.

[59] Sata M, Fukuizumi K, Uchimura Y, et al. Hepatitis C virus infection in patients with clinically diagnosed alcoholic liver diseases. J Viral Hepat 1996;3:143–8.

[60] Ohnishi K, Iida S, Iwama S, et al. The effect of chronic habitual alcohol intake on the development of liver cirrhosis and hepatocellular carcinoma: relation to hepatitis B surface antigen carriage. Cancer 1982;49:672–7.

[61] Fong TL, Kanel GC, Conrad A, et al. Clinical significance of concomitant hepatitis C infection in patients with alcoholic liver disease. Hepatology 1994;19:554–7.

[62] Cromie SL, Jenkins PJ, Bowden DS, et al. Chronic hepatitis C: effect of alcohol on hepatitic activity and viral titre. J Hepatol 1996;25:821–6.

[63] Calle EE, Rodriguez C, Walker-Thurmond K, et al. Overweight, obesity, and mortality from cancer in a prospectively studied cohort of US adults. N Engl J Med 2003;348:1625–38.

[64] Yang S, Lin HZ, Hwang J, et al. Hepatic hyperplasia in noncirrhotic fatty livers: is obesity-related hepatic steatosis a premalignant condition? Cancer Res 2001;61:5016–23.

[65] La Vecchia C, Negri E, Decarli A, et al. Diabetes mellitus and the risk of primary liver cancer. Int J Cancer 1997;73:204–7.

[66] Gillery P, Monboisse JC, Maquart FX, et al. Does oxygen free radical increased formation explain long term complications of diabetes mellitus? Med Hypotheses 1989;29:47–50.

[67] Oberley LW. Free radicals and diabetes. Free Radic Biol Med 1988;5:113–24.

[68] Rosen P, Nawroth PP, King G, et al. The role of oxidative stress in the onset and progression of diabetes and its complications: a summary of a Congress Series sponsored by UNESCO-MCBN, the American Diabetes Association and the German Diabetes Society. Diabetes Metab Res Rev 2001;17:189–212.

[69] Ford ES, Cogswell ME. Diabetes and serum ferritin concentration among US adults. Diabetes Care 1999;22:1978–83.

[70] Du CL, Wang JD. Increased morbidity odds ratio of primary liver cancer and cirrhosis of the liver among vinyl chloride monomer workers. Occup Environ Med 1998;55:528–32.

[71] Evans DM, Williams WJ, Kung IT. Angiosarcoma and hepatocellular carcinoma in vinyl chloride workers. Histopathology 1983;7:377–88.

[72] Mastrangelo G, Fedeli U, Fadda E, et al. Increased risk of hepatocellular carcinoma and liver cirrhosis in vinyl chloride workers: synergistic effect of occupational exposure with alcohol intake. Environ Health Perspect 2004;112:1188–92.

[73] Pirastu R, Belli S, Bruno C, et al. [The mortality among the makers of vinyl chloride in Italy.] Med Lav 1991;82:388–423.

[74] Lieber CS, DeCarli LM. Hepatic microsomal ethanol-oxidizing system. In vitro characteristics and adaptive properties in vivo. J Biol Chem 1970;245:2505–12.

[75] Marion MJ, Boivin-Angele S. Vinyl chloride-specific mutations in humans and animals. IARC Sci Publ 1999;150:315–24.

[76] Marion MJ, De Vivo I, Smith S, et al. The molecular epidemiology of occupational carcinogenesis in vinyl chloride exposed workers. Int Arch Occup Environ Health 1996;68:394–8.

[77] Wang XD, Liu C, Chung J, et al. Chronic alcohol intake reduces retinoic acid concentration and enhances AP-1 (c-Jun and c-Fos) expression in rat liver. Hepatology 1998;28:744–50.

[78] Singletary KW, Barnes SL, van Breemen RB. Ethanol inhibits benzo[a]pyrene-DNA adduct removal and increases 8-oxo-deoxyguanosine formation in human mammary epithelial cells. Cancer Lett 2004;203:139–44.

[79] Parola M, Robino G. Oxidative stress-related molecules and liver fibrosis. J Hepatol 2001;35:297–306.

[80] Aguilar F, Hussain SP, Cerutti P. Aflatoxin B1 induces the transversion of G→T in codon 249 of the p53 tumor suppressor gene in human hepatocytes. Proc Natl Acad Sci USA 1993;90:8586–90.

[81] Bressac B, Kew M, Wands J, et al. Selective G to T mutations of p53 gene in hepatocellular carcinoma from southern Africa. Nature 1991;350:429–31.

[82] Bulatao-Jayme J, Almero EM, Castro CA. A case–control dietary study of primary liver cancer risk from aflatoxin exposure. Int J Epidemiol 1982;11:112–9.

[83] Tuyns AJ. Cancer risks derived from alcohol. Med Oncol Tumor Pharmacother 1987;4:241–4.

[84] del Olmo JA, Serra MA, Rodriguez F, et al. Incidence and risk factors for hepatocellular carcinoma in 967 patients with cirrhosis. J Cancer Res Clin Oncol 1998;124:560–4.

[85] Arico S, Corrao G, Torchio P, et al. A strong negative association between alcohol consumption and the risk of hepatocellular carcinoma in cirrhotic patients. A case–control study. Eur J Epidemiol 1994;10:251–7.

[86] Lands WE. Cellular signals in alcohol-induced liver injury: a review. Alcohol Clin Exp Res 1995;19:928–38.

[87] IARC. I: International Agency for Research on Cancer. Working Group on the evaluation of the carcinogenic risk of chemicals to humans. Acetaldehyde. IARC Monogr 1985;36:101–32.

[88] Clemens DL, Forman A, Jerrells TR, et al. Relationship between acetaldehyde levels and cell survival in ethanol-metabolizing hepatoma cells. Hepatology 2002;35:1196–204.

[89] Beek B, Obe G. Sister chromatid exchanges in human leukocyte chromosomes: spontaneous and induced frequencies in early- and late-proliferating cells in vitro. Hum Genet 1979;49:51–61.

[90] Obe G, Beek B. Mutagenic activity of aldehydes. Drug Alcohol Depend 1979;4:91–4.

[91] Obe G, Ristow H. Mutagenic, cancerogenic and teratogenic effects of alcohol. Mutat Res 1979;65:229–59.

[92] Ristow H, Obe G. Acetaldehyde induces cross-links in DNA and causes sister-chromatid exchanges in human cells. Mutat Res 1978;58:115–9.

[93] Borras E, Coutelle C, Rosell A, et al. Genetic polymorphism of alcohol dehydrogenase in europeans: the ADH2*2 allele decreases the risk for alcoholism and is associated with ADH3*1. Hepatology 2000;31:984–9.

[94] Ohhira M, Fujimoto Y, Matsumoto A, et al. Hepatocellular carcinoma associated with alcoholic liver disease: a clinicopathological study and genetic polymorphism of aldehyde dehydrogenase 2. Alcohol Clin Exp Res 1996;20(9 Suppl):378A–82A.

[95] Shibata A, Fukuda K, Nishiyori A, et al. A case–control study on male hepatocellular carcinoma based on hospital and community controls. J Epidemiol 1998;8:1–5.

[96] Takeshita T, Yang X, Inoue Y, et al. Relationship between alcohol drinking, ADH2 and ALDH2 genotypes, and risk for hepatocellular carcinoma in Japanese. Cancer Lett 2000;149:69–76.

[97] Anderson LM. Modulation of nitrosamine metabolism by ethanol: implications of cancer risk. In: Watson RR, editor. Alcohol and cancer. Boca Raton (FL): CRC Press; 1992. p. 17–54.

[98] Anderson LM, Chhabra SK, Nerurkar PV, et al. Alcohol-related cancer risk: a toxicokinetic hypothesis. Alcohol 1995;12:97–104.

[99] Seitz HK, Osswald BR. Effect of ethanol on procarcinogen activation. In: Watson RR, editor. Alcohol and the gastrointestinal tract. Boca Raton (FL): CRC Press; 1992. p. 55–72.

[100] Ladero JM, Agundez JA, Rodriguez-Lescure A, et al. RsaI polymorphism at the cytochrome P4502E1 locus and risk of hepatocellular carcinoma. Gut 1996;39:330–3.

[101] Tsutsumi M, Takase S, Takada A. Genetic factors related to the development of carcinoma in digestive organs in alcoholics. Alcohol Alcohol Suppl 1993;1B:21–6.

[102] Lee HS, Yoon JH, Kamimura S, et al. Lack of association of cytochrome P450 2E1 genetic polymorphisms with the risk of human hepatocellular carcinoma. Int J Cancer 1997;71:737–40.

[103] Nestmann ER, Bryant DW, Carr CJ. Toxicological significance of DNA adducts: summary of discussions with an expert panel. Regul Toxicol Pharmacol 1996;24:9–18.

[104] Caro AA, Cederbaum AI. Oxidative stress, toxicology, and pharmacology of CYP2E1. Annu Rev Pharmacol Toxicol 2004;44:27–42.

[105] Cederbaum AI. Iron and CYP2E1-dependent oxidative stress and toxicity. Alcohol 2003;30:115–20.

[106] Hoek JB, Pastorino JG. Ethanol, oxidative stress, and cytokine-induced liver cell injury. Alcohol 2002;27:63–8.

[107] Molina PE, Hoek JB, Nelson S, et al. Mechanisms of alcohol-induced tissue injury. Alcohol Clin Exp Res 2003;27:563–75.

[108] Wiley TE, McCarthy M, Breidi L, et al. Impact of alcohol on the histological and clinical progression of hepatitis C infection. Hepatology 1998;28:805–9.

[109] Chung FL, Chen HJ, Nath RG. Lipid peroxidation as a potential endogenous source for the formation of exocyclic DNA adducts. Carcinogenesis 1996;17:2105–11.

[110] el Ghissassi F, Barbin A, Nair J, et al. Formation of 1,N6-ethenoadenine and 3,N4-ethenocytosine by lipid peroxidation products and nucleic acid bases. Chem Res Toxicol 1995; 8:278–83.

[111] Hu W, Feng Z, Eveleigh J, et al. The major lipid peroxidation product, trans-4-hydroxy-2-nonenal, preferentially forms DNA adducts at codon 249 of human p53 gene, a unique mutational hotspot in hepatocellular carcinoma. Carcinogenesis 2002;23:1781–9.

[112] Seitz HK, Suter PM. Ethanol toxicity and nutritional status. In: Cotsones FN, McKay MA, editors. Nutritional toxicology. 2nd ed. London: Taylor and Francis; 2002. p. 122–54.

[113] Gloria L, Cravo M, Camilo ME, et al. Nutritional deficiencies in chronic alcoholics: relation to dietary intake and alcohol consumption. Am J Gastroenterol 1997;92:485–9.

[114] Labadarios D, Rossouw JE, McConnell JB, et al. Vitamin B6 deficiency in chronic liver disease–evidence for increased degradation of pyridoxal-5'-phosphate. Gut 1977;18:23–7.

[115] Lumeng L. The role of acetaldehyde in mediating the deleterious effect of ethanol on pyridoxal 5'-phosphate metabolism. J Clin Invest 1978;62:286–93.

[116] Lumeng L, Li TK. Vitamin B6 metabolism in chronic alcohol abuse. Pyridoxal phosphate levels in plasma and the effects of acetaldehyde on pyridoxal phosphate synthesis and degradation in human erythrocytes. J Clin Invest 1974;53:693–704.

[117] Savage D, Lindenbaum J. Anemia in alcoholics. Medicine (Baltimore) 1986;65:322–38.

[118] Stickel F, Choi SW, Kim YI, et al. Effect of chronic alcohol consumption on total plasma homocysteine level in rats. Alcohol Clin Exp Res 2000;24:259–64.

[119] Vech RL, Lumeng L, Li TK. Vitamin B6 metabolism in chronic alcohol abuse The effect of ethanol oxidation on hepatic pyridoxal 5'-phosphate metabolism. J Clin Invest 1975;55: 1026–32.

[120] Halsted CH, Villanueva JA, Devlin AM, et al. Metabolic interactions of alcohol and folate. J Nutr 2002;132(8 Suppl):2367S–72S.

[121] Ross DM, McMartin KE. Effect of ethanol on folate binding by isolated rat renal brush border membranes. Alcohol 1996;13:449–54.

[122] Purohit V, Russo D. Role of S-adenosyl-L-methionine in the treatment of alcoholic liver disease: introduction and summary of the symposium. Alcohol 2002;27:151–4.

[123] Laufer EM, Hartman TJ, Baer DJ, et al. Effects of moderate alcohol consumption on folate and vitamin B(12) status in postmenopausal women. Eur J Clin Nutr 2004;58(11):1518–24.

[124] Cravo ML, Camilo ME. Hyperhomocysteinemia in chronic alcoholism: relations to folic acid and vitamins B(6) and B(12) status. Nutrition 2000;16:296–302.

[125] Gloria L, Cravo M, Camilo ME, et al. Nutritional deficiencies in chronic alcoholics: relation to dietary intake and alcohol consumption. Am J Gastroenterol 1997;92:485–9.

[126] Lieber CS, Casini A, DeCarli LM, et al. S-adenosyl-L-methionine attenuates alcohol-induced liver injury in the baboon. Hepatology 1990;11:165–72.

[127] Trimble KC, Molloy AM, Scott JM, et al. The effect of ethanol on one-carbon metabolism: increased methionine catabolism and lipotrope methyl-group wastage. Hepatology 1993;18: 984–9.

[128] Bleich S, Degner D, Bandelow B, et al. Plasma homocysteine is a predictor of alcohol withdrawal seizures. Neuroreport 2000;11:2749–52.

[129] Barak AJ, Beckenhauer HC, Hidiroglou N, et al. The relationship of ethanol feeding to the methyl folate trap. Alcohol 1993;10:495–7.

[130] Lieber CS. Alcohol and the liver: 1994 update. Gastroenterology 1994;106:1085–105.

[131] Speisky H, MacDonald A, Giles G, et al. Increased loss and decreased synthesis of hepatic glutathione after acute ethanol administration. Turnover studies. Biochem J 1985;225:565–72.

[132] Brunaud L, Alberto JM, Ayav A, et al. Effects of vitamin B12 and folate deficiencies on DNA methylation and carcinogenesis in rat liver. Clin Chem Lab Med 2003;41:1012–9.

[133] Garro AJ, McBeth DL, Lima V, et al. Ethanol consumption inhibits fetal DNA methylation in mice: implications for the fetal alcohol syndrome. Alcohol Clin Exp Res 1991;15:395–8.

[134] Pogribny IP, James SJ, Jernigan S, et al. Genomic hypomethylation is specific for preneo-

plastic liver in folate/methyl deficient rats and does not occur in non-target tissues. Mutat Res 2004;548:53–9.

[135] Murata H, Tsuji S, Tsujii M, et al. Promoter hypermethylation silences cyclooxygenase-2 (Cox-2) and regulates growth of human hepatocellular carcinoma cells. Lab Invest 2004;84: 1050–9.

[136] Fukai K, Yokosuka O, Chiba T, et al. Hepatocyte growth factor activator inhibitor 2/placental bikunin (HAI-2/PB) gene is frequently hypermethylated in human hepatocellular carcinoma. Cancer Res 2003;63:8674–9.

[137] Okochi O, Hibi K, Sakai M, et al. Methylation-mediated silencing of SOCS-1 gene in hepatocellular carcinoma derived from cirrhosis. Clin Cancer Res 2003;9:5295–8.

[138] Blanchard F, Tracy E, Smith J, et al. DNA methylation controls the responsiveness of hepatoma cells to leukemia inhibitory factor. Hepatology 2003;38:1516–28.

[139] Choi MS, Shim YH, Hwa JY, et al. Expression of DNA methyltransferases in multistep hepatocarcinogenesis. Hum Pathol 2003;34:11–7.

[140] Kondoh N, Hada A, Ryo A, et al. Activation of Galectin-1 gene in human hepatocellular carcinoma involves methylation-sensitive complex formations at the transcriptional upstream and downstream elements. Int J Oncol 2003;23:1575–83.

[141] Lee S, Lee HJ, Kim JH, et al. Aberrant CpG island hypermethylation along multistep hepatocarcinogenesis. Am J Pathol 2003;163:1371–8.

[142] Nagai H, Kim YS, Konishi N, et al. Combined hypermethylation and chromosome loss associated with inactivation of SSI-1/SOCS-1/JAB gene in human hepatocellular carcinomas. Cancer Lett 2002;186:59–65.

[143] Wong CM, Lee JM, Ching YP, et al. Genetic and epigenetic alterations of DLC-1 gene in hepatocellular carcinoma. Cancer Res 2003;63:7646–51.

[144] Yang B, Guo M, Herman JG, et al. Aberrant promoter methylation profiles of tumor suppressor genes in hepatocellular carcinoma. Am J Pathol 2003;163:1101–7.

[145] Yao X, Hu JF, Daniels M, et al. A methylated oligonucleotide inhibits IGF2 expression and enhances survival in a model of hepatocellular carcinoma. J Clin Invest 2003;111:265–73.

[146] Yu J, Ni M, Xu J, et al. Methylation profiling of twenty promoter-CpG islands of genes which may contribute to hepatocellular carcinogenesis. BMC Cancer 2002;2:29.

[147] Yu J, Zhang HY, Ma ZZ, et al. Methylation profiling of twenty four genes and the concordant methylation behaviours of nineteen genes that may contribute to hepatocellular carcinogenesis. Cell Res 2003;13:319–33.

[148] Zhang YJ, Ahsan H, Chen Y, et al. High frequency of promoter hypermethylation of RASSF1A and p16 and its relationship to aflatoxin B1-DNA adduct levels in human hepatocellular carcinoma. Mol Carcinog 2002;35:85–92.

[149] Saffroy R, Pham P, Chiappini F, et al. The MTHFR 677C > T polymorphism is associated with an increased risk of hepatocellular carcinoma in patients with alcoholic cirrhosis. Carcinogenesis 2004;25:1443–8.

[150] Lee SA, Kang D, Nishio H, et al. Methylenetetrahydrofolate reductase polymorphism, diet, and breast cancer in Korean women. Exp Mol Med 2004;36:116–21.

[151] Oyama K, Kawakami K, Maeda K, et al. The association between methylenetetrahydrofolate reductase polymorphism and promoter methylation in proximal colon cancer. Anticancer Res 2004;24:649–54.

[152] Saffroy R, Pham P, Chiappini F, et al. The MTHFR 677C > T polymorphism is associated with an increased risk of hepatocellular carcinoma in patients with alcoholic cirrhosis. Carcinogenesis 2004;25:1443–8.

[153] Zhang J, Zotz RB, Li Y, et al. Methylenetetrahydrofolate reductase C677T polymorphism and predisposition towards esophageal squamous cell carcinoma in a German Caucasian and a northern Chinese population. J Cancer Res Clin Oncol 2004;130(10):57A–80A.

[154] Sun SY, Lotan R. Retinoids and their receptors in cancer development and chemoprevention. Crit Rev Oncol Hematol 2002;41:41–55.

[155] Niles RM. Recent advances in the use of vitamin A (retinoids) in the prevention and treatment of cancer. Nutrition 2000;16:1084–9.

[156] Niles RM. Vitamin A and cancer. Nutrition 2000;16:573–6.

[157] Rodriguez-Leon J, Merino R, Macias D, et al. Retinoic acid regulates programmed cell death through BMP signalling. Nat Cell Biol 1999;1:125–6.

[158] Dragnev KH, Petty WJ, Dmitrovsky E. Retinoid targets in cancer therapy and chemoprevention. Cancer Biol Ther 2003;2(4 Suppl):S150–6.

[159] Fraser PD, Bramley PM. The biosynthesis and nutritional uses of carotenoids. Prog Lipid Res 2004;43:228–65.

[160] Freemantle SJ, Spinella MJ, Dmitrovsky E. Retinoids in cancer therapy and chemoprevention: promise meets resistance. Oncogene 2003;22:7305–15.

[161] Johanning GL, Piyathilake CJ. Retinoids and epigenetic silencing in cancer. Nutr Rev 2003; 61:284–9.

[162] Pryor WA, Stahl W, Rock CL. Beta carotene: from biochemistry to clinical trials. Nutr Rev 2000;58(2 pt 1):39–53.

[163] Leo MA, Lieber CS. Hepatic vitamin A depletion in alcoholic liver injury. N Engl J Med 1982; 307:597–601.

[164] Leo MA, Lieber CS. Alcohol, vitamin A, and beta-carotene: adverse interactions, including hepatotoxicity and carcinogenicity. Am J Clin Nutr 1999;69:1071–85.

[165] Seitz HK. Alcohol and retinoid metabolism. Gut 2000;47:748–50.

[166] Wang XD. Retinoids and alcohol-related carcinogenesis. J Nutr 2003;133:287S–90S.

[167] Liu C, Russell RM, Seitz HK, et al. Ethanol enhances retinoic acid metabolism into polar metabolites in rat liver via induction of cytochrome P4502E1. Gastroenterology 2001;120: 179–89.

[168] Chung J, Liu C, Smith DE, et al. Restoration of retinoic acid concentration suppresses ethanol-enhanced c-Jun expression and hepatocyte proliferation in rat liver. Carcinogenesis 2001;22:1213–9.

[169] Walker PR, Saas P, Dietrich PY. Tumor expression of Fas ligand (CD95L) and the consequences. Curr Opin Immunol 1998;10:564–72.

[170] Huang J, Cai MY, Wei DP. HLA class I expression in primary hepatocellular carcinoma. World J Gastroenterol 2002;8:654–7.

[171] Villunger A, Strasser A. The great escape: is immune evasion required for tumor progression? Nat Med 1999;5:874–5.

[172] Diefenbach A, Raulet DH. The innate immune response to tumors and its role in the induction of T-cell immunity. Immunol Rev 2002;188(3 Suppl 7):5–11.

[173] Foss FM. Immunologic mechanisms of antitumor activity. Semin Oncol 2002;29(3 Suppl 7): 5–11.

[174] Khong HT, Restifo NP. Natural selection of tumor variants in the generation of "tumor escape" phenotypes. Nat Immunol 2002;3:999–1005.

[175] Kiessling R, Pawelec G, Welsh RM, et al. Have tumor cells learnt from microorganisms how to fool the immune system? Escape from immune surveillance of tumors and microorganisms: emerging mechanisms and shared strategies. Mol Med Today 2000;6:344–6.

[176] Cook RT. Alcohol abuse, alcoholism, and damage to the immune system—a review. Alcohol Clin Exp Res 1998;22:1927–42.

[177] Wu WJ, Pruett SB. Suppression of splenic natural killer cell activity in a mouse model for binge drinking. I. Direct effects of ethanol and its major metabolites are not primarily responsible for decreased natural killer cell activity. J Pharmacol Exp Ther 1996;278:1325–30.

[178] Taylor AN, Ben Eliyahu S, Yirmiya R, et al. Actions of alcohol on immunity and neoplasia in fetal alcohol exposed and adult rats. Alcohol Alcohol Suppl 1993;2:69–74.

[179] Wu WJ, Pruett SB. Ethanol decreases host resistance to pulmonary metastases in a mouse model: role of natural killer cells and the ethanol-induced stress response. Int J Cancer 1999; 82:886–92.

[180] Roselle G, Mendenhall CL, Grossmann C. Effects of alcohol on immunity and cancer. In: Yirmiya R, Taylor AN, editors. Alcohol, immunity and cancer. Boca Raton (FL): CRC Press; 1993. p. 3–22.

CLINICS IN
LIVER DISEASE

Clin Liver Dis 9 (2005) 171–181

Liver Transplantation for Alcoholic Liver Disease

Rowen K. Zetterman, MD, MACP, FACG[a,b,*]

[a]Nebraska-Western Iowa VA Health Care System, 4101 Woolworth Avenue, Omaha, NE 68105, USA
[b]University of Nebraska Medical Center, 983332 Nebraska Medical Center, Omaha,
NE 68198-3332, USA

Although alcohol does not produce end-stage liver disease in all chronic alcoholics, it can lead to severe liver injury such as alcoholic hepatitis or cirrhosis, sometimes in conjunction with other injurious factors such as concomitant chronic hepatitis C virus (HCV) infection [1]. In the past, therapy for alcoholic cirrhosis was limited to the control of complications of portal hypertension. With the advent of orthotopic liver transplantation, however, replacement of the diseased liver has become an acceptable option of treatment of alcoholic cirrhosis and its complications [2–9]. When compared with simulation models and a cohort of alcoholic cirrhosis patients not accepted for transplantation, transplanted alcoholic liver disease patients have a longer overall survival [10], providing evidence of the efficacy of liver transplantation for end-stage alcoholic liver disease.

Despite the reported successes in transplantation of patients with alcoholic cirrhosis, there are still issues to be resolved. Whether patients who have ongoing alcoholic hepatitis [11] or those continuing to consume ethanol [12] are acceptable candidates remains to be settled. In this review, we address candidacy, posttransplant recidivism, and postoperative care of patients transplanted for end-stage alcoholic liver disease, but will not review in detail the comorbidity pre- or posttransplantation for those with both alcohol and HCV.

* Nebraska-Western Iowa VA Health Care System, 4101 Woolworth Avenue, Omaha, NE 68105.
E-mail address: rzetterm@unmc.edu

Pretransplant social issues

There are some who feel that patients with end-stage alcoholic liver disease are unworthy candidates for liver transplantation because they have personal responsibility for the cause of their liver disease [13,14]. Even if considered for transplantation, it has been suggested that alcoholic patients should have a lower priority for receipt of a cadaver donor liver than others [15–17]. This attitude is compounded by other social issues such as the higher unemployment status of patients with alcoholic liver disease when compared with the pretransplantation status of patients with other types of end-stage liver disease [18]. Fortunately, these issues are dissipating as points of public concern as posttransplantation data confirm that the patient with alcoholic liver disease tends to do well following liver transplantation [2] and returns to work as frequently as other liver recipients.

There are still some concerns about organ donation that remain. Some potential donors believe that alcoholics are unworthy recipients, and as a consequence, these persons say they will not donate their loved one's organs on the chance they would go an alcoholic [19]. These stigmas about alcoholism and its attendant social issues may even affect the willingness of living-related donation [20]. No matter what the issue, it is clear that we all need to work at enhancing donation, in general, using creative ideas to improve fairness of donation and allocation [21].

Candidate selection

Although specific candidate selection criteria differ from program to program [22], patients with alcoholic liver disease are transplanted in virtually all programs in the United States. I recommend that patients should be referred for evaluation as soon as complications such as variceal hemorrhage, ascites, or hepatic encephalopathy develop. Complications of hypersplenism should also be considered an indication for early referral, as hypersplenism in the presence of decompensated alcoholic cirrhosis is associated with a greater likelihood of subsequent spontaneous bacterial peritonitis and variceal hemorrhage [23]. As a rule of thumb, it is better to refer patients too early for liver transplantation than too late when transplantation is no longer an option because of the associated severity of illness. The transplant center can also assist the clinician with decisions of whether liver transplantation or surgical shunting will be the most appropriate plan for the patient with variceal hemorrhage or whether short-term placement of a transvenous intrahepatic portosystemic shunt might allow sufficient time to improve the patient's chances for subsequent transplantation.

Each patient should also be carefully evaluated for other risk factors such as HCV. When patients with HCV are evaluated for liver transplantation, a careful history will identify that up to 35% will have a history of excessive ethanol ingestion [24]. Other associated disorders of alcoholism may also lead to transplantation. Two alcoholic patients have been transplanted as a consequence of acute hepatotoxicity from disulfiram [25,26].

Perhaps the most difficult and still unresolved issue in the transplantation of alcoholic patients is what to do with the patient with alcoholic hepatitis. At present, most programs still refuse to transplant those with acute, decompensated alcoholic hepatitis. I suspect this issue will continue to be debated, as the presence of alcoholic hepatitis does not predict an increased likelihood of recidivism [27]. Furthermore, the overall outcome of liver transplantation of patients with alcoholic hepatitis may be similar to patients with end-stage alcoholic liver disease lacking evidence of alcoholic hepatitis [27]. As the complications of some alcoholic patient's liver disease will stabilize with abstinence and not result in urgent liver transplantation, I believe it is acceptable to use a required period of abstinence that also prevents liver transplantation of the patient with alcoholic hepatitis.

A multidisciplinary team including a psychologist and psychiatrist should carefully evaluate each patient with alcoholic cirrhosis being considered for liver transplantation [28,29]. A psychiatrist is an important constituent of the team, as those with substance abuse have been identified to have more distress, less adaptive behavior skills, and more character pathology [30]. Such careful evaluation preoperatively can also assist with planning and care after transplantation when psychiatric issues and recidivism may resurface.

Although some have questioned the reliability of an alcoholic patient's history of alcohol consumption, at least one study indicates that such history obtained at the time of consideration of liver transplantation tends to be reliable [31]. The specific criteria used to determine candidacy typically includes a period of sobriety [32]. The American Association for the Study of Liver Diseases guideline suggests it should be at least 6 months [33], and this interval is commonly used by many centers. Despite such recommendations, however, there is little evidence that length of pretransplant sobriety correlates with the likelihood of posttransplant recidivism [34,35]. Some programs have also indicated that patients must go through outpatient treatment programs or attend and document attendance at Alcoholics Anonymous meetings. Whether to mandate alcoholism treatment is not clear in all cases. Many patients with advanced alcoholic liver disease are too ill to successfully undergo such therapy. In addition, end-stage alcoholic cirrhosis patients tend to have less alcohol craving and are also less motivated to undergo treatment. I believe that the most important issue to assess in the end-stage patient with alcoholic cirrhosis is whether they have any insight into the cause of their liver disease as those who understand how they got to their current status are more likely to remain abstinent following liver transplantation than those who do not [36].

Liver transplantation

Although patients with end-stage alcoholic liver disease tend to have more advanced clinical liver disease at transplantation than patients transplanted for other end-stage liver diseases [37,38], the early outcome of patient with alcoholic cirrhosis including resource use and retransplantation rate is similar to that of other liver diseases [39]. A worsened outcome has been reported for those alcoholic cirrhosis patients over 50 years of age who tend to have a longer initial hospitalization posttransplantation and a higher risk of early mortality [40]. Long-term psychologic and physical health for survivors is good [41].

General

In planning postoperative care, it is important to establish short-term and long-term programs to support continued abstinence [42]. In addition, the pretransplant psychologic/psychiatric evaluation should be reviewed to determine what additional therapy and support systems may be needed for the patient. Some pretransplant problems such as spur cell anemia [43] and polyneuropathy [44] will resolve following liver transplantation, while others such as hypersplenism often persist. Cognitive function may also improve following transplantation of the alcoholic, although memory typically does not [45].

Alcoholic patients transplanted for end-stage liver disease have been reported to develop an acute postoperative confusional state lasting up to 3 days [46]. An association of the confusional state with a shorter pretransplantation interval of sobriety and higher blood ammonia levels at the time of transplantation was noted in these patients. The mechanism of the confusional state is unclear, and supportive care is recommended. Although it will resolve, it may contribute to a longer initial length of hospital stay.

Those transplanted for end-stage alcoholic liver disease have a greater prevalence of posttransplant diabetes mellitus [47] and often require initial insulin therapy. Intensive insulin management early during posttransplant care is crucial, and can contribute to a reduction of both intensive care and hospital length of stay. Bacterial infections also are more frequent in the alcoholic after transplantation [28,48], although viral infections such as cytomegalovirus may or may not be more common than in other liver diseases [39,49,50].

Survival

The initial survival of patients transplanted for end-stage alcoholic liver disease is excellent [12,36,37,49,51–60], and appears to be unaffected by the return of the patient to modest drinking [40,52,53]. Furthermore, early postoperative clinical health is as good for the alcoholic as for patients with other liver diseases posttransplantation [61]. There is some evidence that longer pretransplant abstinence may improve long-term posttransplant outcomes [53]. When long-term outcomes were assessed using the United Network of Organ Sharing database, the overall long-term outcome for the alcoholic may be poorer, in part explained by the greater severity of pretransplant illness [62] and an increase in late complications such as tumors, infections, and age-related disease [63].

Recurrent disease

With a return to drinking ethanol posttransplantation, recurrent alcoholic liver disease can develop [64], and typically includes fatty liver [52,65] and pericellular fibrosis [52]. As most patients do not return to the severity of drinking they experienced pretransplantation, recurrent end-stage liver disease is uncommon, although alcoholic hepatitis and cirrhosis have been reported [25,66]. In addition, graft loss from recidivism is uncommon [60,63]. Nonspecific hepatitis can develop in the graft of patients transplanted for alcoholic liver disease but is similar in frequency and severity to that of those transplanted for other diseases [67].

Allograft cellular rejection

Although not reported by all studies [39,67], it has been suggested that acute cellular rejection is less likely in the alcoholic than the nonalcoholic patient following orthotopic liver transplantation [47,48,68]. This reduced risk of allograft rejection is consistent with our program's experience, and suggests that the alcoholic patient is intrinsically immunosuppressed. A return to consumption of ethanol may or may not further reduce the risk of acute cellular rejection [67,69]. Similarly, the development of chronic rejection in those with alcoholic liver disease also appears to be less [48,63,70], and may be further reduced in likelihood by ethanol consumption [69]. The role of concomitant HCV infection and its relationship to the development of acute and chronic allograft rejection in those with alcoholic liver disease remains to be determined.

Posttransplant social issues

Recidivism

A return to ethanol consumption following liver transplantation is considered a serious problem for most liver transplant programs. Unfortunately, there may be few clues to its occurrence. Although liver tests are routinely followed in all transplant patients, these tests are a poor indicator of recidivism [71,72]. Detection of carbohydrate-deficient transferrin levels has been proposed as a marker of alcohol consumption [73], although it does not appear to be reliable [34,74].

Although patients transplanted for end-stage alcoholic liver disease typically drink less ethanol than they did pretransplantation [75], recidivism is prevalent and ranges from 8% to 33% of patients [36,50,52,53,60,64,76–82]. Most studies indicate that it is not related to the length of pretransplant sobriety [54,60,63]. However, the association of recidivism with shorter intervals of pretransplantation sobriety in some studies [49,75,83,84] has given credence to the use of a minimum of 6 months sobriety pretransplantation for most programs including our own. It is of interest that patients transplanted with acute alcoholic hepatitis, and consequently a shorter interval of pretransplantation sobriety, does not cause an unequivocal likelihood of recidivism [27,66]. In general, the prevalence of drinking among alcoholic liver disease patients posttransplantation is similar to those transplanted for other liver diseases [75,82]. Perhaps most surprisingly, it is unclear that subsequent ethanol consumption by the transplantation recipient has any significant effect on long-term outcome [76].

Many studies have attempted to identify the factors that contribute to a greater likelihood of recidivism. In general, fostering candor between the transplant team and the alcoholic patient seems crucial to care and a reduction of recidivism [85]. In addition, I feel that a patient who has good insight to the relationship of alcoholism to their liver disease and other social problems is more likely to remain abstinent than those who fail to have adequate insight [36]. The clues that should alert the transplantation team to a high risk of recidivism include a family history of alcoholism [86]; poor living arrangements associated with a history of suicide ideation; failure or refusal to participate in ethanol rehabilitation and a history of prior hospitalization for alcoholism [87]; use of other forms of substance abuse [88]; an earlier age for the initial onset of drinking [83]; male gender plus an inadequate social environment [49]; female gender and unemployment [89]; and those alcoholics with dual diagnosis [30]. In general, all these factors can be identified before liver transplantation of the alcoholic and can help to tailor postoperative care so as to reduce recidivism.

Compliance

Although raised initially as an issue of concern, compliance is rarely an issue in the postoperative care of the patients transplanted for alcoholic liver disease [72,78]. Medication use, attendance at medical visits, and general compliance are typically good and unaffected by recidivism, even if it should develop [53,79,90]. Motivation including insight and readiness for treatment coupled with compliance for health care seems associated with continued abstinence [91].

Quality of life

Studies are conflicting on the frequency with which those transplanted for end-stage alcoholic liver disease return to work upon recovery. Some studies report it as less [53,82] while others say it is as good as for those transplanted for nonalcoholic liver disease [18,28,92,93]. For all, the quality of life typically improves posttransplantation [18,83], in conjunction with good social rehabilitation, although there is a greater likelihood of posttransplantation marital separation [47].

Special issues

Tumors

Skin and hematologic cancers are increased in prevalence in all patients following liver transplantation. Solid tumors are generally squamous cell in type, although those with predisposing conditions such as ulcerative colitis have an increased risk of colorectal cancer when transplanted for sclerosing cholangitis. In one study, the general risk of solid tumors following liver transplantation was more than 5% [94], while those transplanted for alcoholic liver disease were at even greater risk of squamous cell carcinomas of the oropharynx, esophagus, lung, and vulva [60,63,94–96]. Ongoing surveillance with periodic dental and pharyngeal examinations, pap smears where appropriate, and careful follow-up of new respiratory and esophageal symptoms is mandatory.

Osteopenia

All liver patients are at an increased risk of hepatic osteodystrophy, and it typically worsens the first year posttransplant as a consequence of corticosteroids and nutritional issues [97,98]. Patients transplanted for alcoholic liver disease have an increased fracture risk in part due to alcoholism [99], with up to 17% reporting fractures (often lumbar spine) during the first year postoperative.

Summary

Patients with end-stage alcoholic liver disease should be considered for liver transplantation. A careful pretransplant evaluation must be undertaken to assess for both medical and psychiatric factors that will continue to require attention following transplantation. Although most programs require at least 6 months of ethanol abstinence before consideration of liver transplantation, there is little evidence that this conclusively predicts a reduction in recidivism. Most programs continue to exclude those with alcoholic hepatitis. Postoperatively, attention to psychiatric issues, recidivism, compliance, and assessment for tumors, especially squamous cell carcinomas, should be undertaken.

References

[1] Maddrey WC. Alcohol-induced liver disease. Clin Liver Dis 2000;4:115–31.
[2] Starzl TE, Van Thiel D, Tzakis AG, et al. Orthotopic liver transplantation for alcoholic liver disease. JAMA 1988;260:2542–4.
[3] Van Thiel DH, Carr B, Iwatsuki S, et al. Liver transplantation for alcoholic liver disease, viral hepatitis and hepatic neoplasms. Transplant Proc 1991;23:1917–21.

[4] Kumar S, Stauber RE, Gavaler JS, et al. Orthotopic liver transplantation for alcoholic liver disease. Hepatology 1990;11:159–64.

[5] Morgan MY. The prognosis and outcome of alcoholic liver disease. Alcohol Alcohol Suppl 1994;2:335–43.

[6] Tome S, Lucey MR. Review article: current management of alcoholic liver disease. Aliment Pharmacol Ther 2004;19:707–14.

[7] Walsh K, Alexander G. Alcoholic liver disease. Postgrad Med J 2000;76:280–6.

[8] Hill DB, Kugelmas M. Alcoholic liver disease: treatment strategies for the potentially reversible stages. Postgrad Med 1998;103:261–75.

[9] Lucey MR. Liver transplantation for alcoholic liver disease. Baillieres Clin Gastroenterol 1993;7:717–27.

[10] Poynard T, Naveau S, Doffoel M, et al. Evaluation of efficacy of liver transplantation in alcoholic cirrhosis using matched and simulated controls: 5-year survival. J Hepatol 1999;30:1130–7.

[11] Haber PS, Warner R, Seth D, et al. Pathogenesis and management of alcoholic hepatitis. J Gastroenterol Hepatol 2003;18:1332–44.

[12] Gledhill J, Burroughs A, Rolles K, et al. Psychiatric and social outcome following liver transplantation for alcoholic liver disease: a controlled study. J Psychosom Res 1999;46:359–68.

[13] Martens W. Do alcoholic liver transplantation candidates merit lower medical priority than non-alcoholic candidates? Transpl Int 2001;14:170–5.

[14] Beresford T. The limits of philosophy in liver transplantation. Transpl Int 2001;14:176–9.

[15] Neuberger J. Transplantation for alcoholic liver disease: a perspective from Europe. Liver Transpl Surg 1998;5(Suppl 1):S51–7.

[16] Glannon W. Responsibility, alcoholism, and transplantation. J Med Philos 1998;23:31–49.

[17] Moss AH, Siegler M. Should alcoholics compete equally for liver transplantation. JAMA 1991; 265:1295–8.

[18] Bravata DM, Keeffe EB. Quality of life and employment after liver transplantation. Liver Trans 2001;7(11 Suppl 1):S119–23.

[19] Ubel PA, Jepson C, Baron J, et al. Allocation of transplantable organs: do people want to punish patients for causing their illness? Liver Transpl 2001;7:600–7.

[20] Rudow DL, Russo MW, Hafliger S, et al. Clinical and ethnic differences in candidates listed for liver transplantation with and without potential living donors. Liver Transpl 2003;9:254–9.

[21] Surman OS, Cosimi AB. Ethical dichotomies in organ transplantation. A time for bridge building. Gen Hosp Psychiatry 1996;18(6 Suppl):13S–9S.

[22] Snyder SL, Drooker M, Strain JJ. A survey estimate of academic liver transplant teams' selection practices for alcohol-dependent applicants. Psychosomatics 1996;37:432–7.

[23] Liangpunsakul S, Ulmer BJ, Chalasani N. Predictors and implications of severe hypersplenism in patients with cirrhosis. Am J Med Sci 2003;326:111–6.

[24] Levy MT, Chen JJ, McGuinness PH, et al. Liver transplantation for hepatitis C-associated cirrhosis in a single Australian centre: referral patterns and transplant outcomes. J Gastroenterol Hepatol 1997;12:453–9.

[25] Mohanty SR, La Brecque DR, Mitros FA, et al. Liver transplantation for disulfiram-induced hepatic failure. J Clin Gastroenterol 2004;38:292–5.

[26] Rabkin JM, Corless CL, Orloff SL, et al. Liver transplantation for disulfiram-induced liver failure. Am J Gastroenterol 1998;93:830–1.

[27] Tome S, Martinez-Ray C, Gonzalez-Quintela A, et al. Influence of superimposed alcoholic hepatitis on the outcome of liver transplantation for end-stage alcoholic liver disease. J Hepatol 2002;36:793–8.

[28] Zibari GB, Edwin D, Wall L, et al. Liver transplantation for alcoholic liver disease. Clin Transplant 1996;10:676–9.

[29] Stilley CS, Miller DJ, Gayowski T, et al. Psychological characteristics for liver transplantation: differences according to history of substance abuse and UNOS listing. J Clin Psychol 1999; 55:1287–97.

[30] Tripp LE, Clemons JR, Goldstein RR, et al. Drinking patterns in liver transplant recipients. Psychosomatics 1996;37:249–53.

[31] Yates WR, Labrecque DR, Pfab D. The reliability of alcoholism history in patients with alcohol-related cirrhosis. Alcohol Alcohol 1998;33:488–94.

[32] Krom RA. Liver transplantation and alcohol: who should get transplants? Hepatology 1994; 20:28S–32S.

[33] Lucey MR, Brown KA, Everson GT, et al. Minimal criteria for placement of adults on the liver transplant waiting list: a report of a national conference organized by the American Society of Transplant Physicians and the American Association for the Study of Liver Diseases. Liver Transpl Surg 1997;3:628–37.

[34] DiMartini A, Jain A, Irish W, et al. Outcome of liver transplantation in critically ill patients with alcoholic cirrhosis: survival according to medical variables and sobriety. Transplantation 1998; 66:298–302.

[35] Yates WR, Martin M, Labrecque D, et al. A model to examine the validity of the 6-month abstinence criterion for liver transplantation. Alcohol Clin Exp Res 1998;22:513–7.

[36] Burra P, Mioni D, Cilio U, et al. Long-term medical and psycho-social evaluation of patients undergoing orthotopic liver transplantation for alcoholic liver disease. Transpl Int 2000; 13(Suppl 1):S174–8.

[37] Yerdel MA, Gunson B, Mirza D, et al. Portal vein thrombosis in adults undergoing liver transplantation: risk factors, screening, management, and outcome. Transplantation 2000;69: 1873–81.

[38] Stell DA, McAlister VC, Thorburn D. A comparison of disease severity and survival rates after liver transplantation in the United Kingdom, Canada, and the United States. Liver Transpl 2004; 10:898–902.

[39] McCurry KR, Baliga P, Merion RM, et al. Resource utilization and outcome of liver transplantation for alcoholic cirrhosis. A case–control study. Arch Surg 1992;127:772–6.

[40] Gerhardt TC, Goldstein RM, Urschel HC, et al. Alcohol use after liver transplantation for alcoholic cirrhosis. Transplantation 1996;62:1060–3.

[41] Beresford TP, Schwartz J, Wilson D, et al. The short-term psychological health of alcoholic and non-alcoholic liver transplant recipients. Alcohol Clin Exp Res 1992;16:996–1000.

[42] DiMarini A, Weinrieb R, Fireman M. Liver transplantation in patients with alcohol and other substance use disorders. Psychiatr Clin N Am 2002;25:195–209.

[43] Malik P, Bogetti D, Sileri P, et al. Spur cell anemia in alcoholic cirrhosis: cure by orthotopic liver transplantation and recurrence after liver graft failure. Int Surg 2002;87:201–4.

[44] Spahn TW, Lohse AW, Otto G, et al. Remission of severe alcoholic polyneuropathy after liver transplantation. Z Gastroenterol 1995;33:711–4.

[45] Aria AM, Tarter RE, Starzl TE, et al. Improvement in cognitive functioning of alcoholics following liver transplantation. Alcohol Clin Exp Res 1991;15:956–62.

[46] Buis CI, Wiesner RH, Krom RA, et al. Acute confusional state following liver transplantation for alcoholic liver disease. Neurology 2002;59:601–5.

[47] Abosh D, Rosser B, Kaita K, et al. Outcomes following liver transplantation for patients with alcohol-versus nonalcohol-induced liver disease. Can J Gastroenterol 2000;14:851–5.

[48] Farges O, Saliba F, Farhamant H, et al. Incidence of rejection and infection after liver transplantation as a function of primary disease: possible influence of alcohol and polyclonal immunoglobulins. Hepatology 1996;23:240–8.

[49] Platz KP, Mueller AR, Spree E, et al. Liver transplantation for alcoholic cirrhosis. Transpl Int 2000;13(Suppl 1):S127–30.

[50] Stefanini GF, Biselli M, Grazi GL, et al. Orthotopic liver transplantation for alcoholic liver disease: rates of survival, complications and relapse. Hepatogastroenterology 1997;44:1356–9.

[51] Osorio RW, Friese CE, Ascher NL, et al. Orthotopic liver transplantation for end-stage alcoholic liver disease. Transpl Proc 1993;25:1133–4.

[52] Burra P, Mioni D, Cecchetto A, et al. Histological features after liver transplantation in alcoholic cirrhotics. J Hepatol 2001;34:716–22.

[53] Pageaux GP, Michel J, Coste V, et al. Alcoholic cirrhosis is a good indication for liver transplantation, even for case of recidivism. Gut 1999;45:421–6.

[54] Mackie J, Groves K, Hoyle A, et al. Orthotopic liver transplantation of alcoholic liver disease:

a retrospective analysis of survival, recidivism, and risk factors predisposing to recidivism. Liver Transpl 2001;7:418–27.

[55] Goldar-Najafi A, Gordon FD, Lewis WD, et al. Liver transplantation for alcoholic liver disease with or without hepatitis C. Int J Surg Pathol 2002;10:115–22.

[56] Dhar S, Omran L, Bacon BR, et al. Liver transplantation in patients with chronic hepatitis C and alcoholism. Dig Dis Sci 1999;44:2003–7.

[57] Bird GL, O'Grady JG, Harvey FA, et al. Liver transplantation in patients with alcoholic cirrhosis: selection criteria and rates of survival and relapse. BMJ 1990;301:15–7.

[58] Anand AC, Ferraz-Neto BH, Nightingale P, et al. Liver transplantation for alcoholic liver disease: evaluation of a selection protocol. Hepatology 1997;25:1478–84.

[59] De Maria N, Colantoni A, Van Thiel DH. Liver transplantation for alcoholic liver disease. Hepatogastroenterology 1998;45:1364–8.

[60] Bellamy CO, DiMartini AM, Ruppert K, et al. Liver transplantation for alcoholic cirrhosis: long term follow-up and impact of disease recurrence. Transplantation 2001;72:619–26.

[61] Knechtle SJ, Fleming MF, Barry KL, et al. Liver transplantation for alcoholic liver disease. Surgery 1992;112:694–701.

[62] Roberts MS, Angus DC, Bryce CL, et al. Survival after liver transplantation in the United States: a disease-specific analysis of the UNOS database. Liver Transpl 2004;10:886–97.

[63] Jain A, DiMartini A, Kashyap R, et al. Long-term follow-up after liver transplantation for alcoholic liver disease under tacrolimus. Transplantation 2000;70:1335–42.

[64] Yusoff IF, House AK, De Boer WB, et al. Disease recurrence after liver transplantation in Western Australia. J Gastroenterol Hepatol 2002;17:203–7.

[65] Tang H, Boulton R, Gunson B, et al. Patterns of alcohol consumption after liver transplantation. Gut 1998;43:140–5.

[66] Conjeevaram HS, Hart J, Lissoos TW, et al. Rapidly progressive liver injury and fatal alcoholic hepatitis occurring after liver transplantation in alcoholic patients. Transplantation 1999;67:1562–8.

[67] Lucey MR, Carr K, Beresford TP, et al. Alcohol use after liver transplantation in alcoholics: a clinical cohort follow-up study. Hepatology 1997;25:1223–7.

[68] Bathgate AJ, Hynd P, Sommerville D, et al. The prediction of acute cellular rejection in orthotopic liver transplantation. Liver Transpl Surg 1999;5:475–9.

[69] Van Thiel DH, Bonet H, Gavaler J, et al. Effect of alcohol use on allograft rejection rates after liver transplantation for alcoholic liver disease. Alcohol Clin Exp Res 1995;19:1151–5.

[70] Berlakovich GA, Steininger R, Herbst F, et al. Efficacy of liver transplantation for alcoholic cirrhosis with respect to recidivism and compliance. Transplantation 1994;58:560–5.

[71] Rommelspacher H, Wiest M, Neuhaus R, et al. Long-term changes of markers of alcoholism after orthotopic liver transplantation (OLT). Transplantation 1996;62:1451–5.

[72] Berlakovich GA, Steininger R, Herbst F, et al. Transplantation for alcoholic cirrhosis: how does recurrence of disease harm the graft? Transpl Int 1994;7(Suppl 1):S123–7.

[73] Berlakovich BA, Windhager T, Freundorfer E, et al. Carbohydrate deficient transferrin for the detection of alcohol relapse after orthotopic liver transplantation for alcoholic cirrhosis. Transplantation 1999;67:1231–5.

[74] Heinemann A, Sterneck M, Kuhlencordt R, et al. Carbohydrate-deficient transferrin: diagnostic efficacy among patients with end-stage liver disease before and after liver transplantation. Alcohol Clin Exp Res 1998;22:1806–12.

[75] Pereira SP, Howard LM, Mulesan P, et al. Quality of life after liver transplantation for alcoholic cirrhosis. Liver Transpl 2000;6:762–8.

[76] Beresford TP, Martin B, Alfers J. Developing a brief monitoring procedure for alcohol-dependent graft recipients. Psychosomatics 2004;45:220–3.

[77] Pageaux GP, Bismuth M, Perney P, et al. Alcohol relapse after liver transplantation for alcoholic liver disease: does it matter? J Hepatol 2003;38:629–34.

[78] Gish RG, Lee A, Brooks L, et al. Long-term follow-up of patients diagnosed with alcohol dependence or alcohol abuse who were evaluated for liver transplantation. Liver Transpl 2001;7:581–7.

[79] Berlakovich GA, Langer F, Freundorfer E, et al. General compliance after liver transplantation for alcoholic cirrhosis. Transpl Int 2000;13:129–35.

[80] Campbell DA, McGee JC, Punch JD, et al. One center's experience with liver transplantation: alcohol use relapse over the long-term. Liver Transpl Surg 1998;4(Suppl 1):S58–64.

[81] Osorio RW, Ascher NL, Avery M, et al. Predicting recidivism after orthotopic liver transplantation for alcoholic liver disease. Hepatology 1994;20:105–10.

[82] Keeffe EB, Esquivel CO. Controversies in patient selection for liver transplantation. West J Med 1993;159:586–93.

[83] Bravata DM, Olkin I, Barnato AE, et al. Employment and alcohol use after liver transplantation for alcoholic and nonalcoholic liver disease: a systematic review. Liver Transpl 2001;7: 191–203.

[84] Foster PF, Fabrega F, Karademir S, et al. Prediction of abstinence from ethanol in alcoholic recipients following liver transplantation. Hepatology 1997;25:1469–77.

[85] Weinrieb RM, Van Horn DH, McLellan AT, et al. Interpreting the significance of drinking by alcohol-dependent liver transplant patients: fostering candor is the key to recovery. Liver Transpl 2000;6:769–76.

[86] Jauhar S, Talwalkar JA, Schneekloth T, et al. Analysis of factors that predict alcohol relapse following liver transplantation. Liver Transpl 2004;10:408–11.

[87] Karman JF, Sileri P, Kamuda D, et al. Risk factors for failure to meet listing requirements in liver transplant candidates with alcoholic cirrhosis. Transplantation 2001;71:1210–3.

[88] DiMartini A, Day N, Dew MA, et al. Alcohol use following liver transplantation: a comparison of follow-up methods. Psychosomatics 2001;42:55–62.

[89] Tringali RA, Trzepacz PT, DiMartini A, et al. Assessment and follow-up of alcohol-dependent liver transplantation patients. A clinical cohort. Gen Hosp Psychiatry 1996;18(6 Suppl):70S–7S.

[90] Fabrega E, Crespo J, Casafont F, et al. Alcoholic recidivism after liver transplantation for alcoholic cirrhosis. J Clin Gastroenterol 1998;26:204–6.

[91] Roggla H, Roggla G, Muhlbacher F. Psychiatric prognostic factors in patients with alcohol-related end-stage liver disease before liver transplantation. Wien Klin Wochenschr 1996;108: 272–5.

[92] Cowling T, Jennings LW, Goldstein RM, et al. Societal reintegration after liver transplantation: findings in alcohol-related and nonalcohol-related transplant recipients. Ann Surg 2004; 239:93–8.

[93] Cowling T, Jennings LW, Jung GS, et al. Comparing quality of life following liver transplantation for Laennec's versus non-Laennec's patients. Clin Transplant 2000;14:115–20.

[94] Benloch S, Berenguer M, Prieto M, et al. De novo internal neoplasms after liver transplantation: increased risk and aggressive behavior in recent years? Am J Transplant 2004;4:596–604.

[95] Kenngott S, Gerbes AL, Schaure R, et al. Rapid development of esophageal squamous cell carcinoma after liver transplantation for alcohol-induced cirrhosis. Transpl Int 2003;16:639–41.

[96] Duvoux C, Delacroix I, Richardjet JP, et al. Increased incidence of oropharyngeal squamous cell carcinomas after liver transplantation for alcoholic cirrhosis. Transplantation 1999;67:418–21.

[97] Ng TM, Bajjoka IE. Treatment options for osteoporosis in chronic liver disease patients requiring liver transplantation. Ann Pharmacother 1999;33:233–5.

[98] Carey EJ, Balan V, Kremers WK, et al. Osteopenia and osteoporosis in patients with end-stage liver disease caused by hepatitis C and alcoholic liver disease: not just a cholestatic problem. Liver Transpl 2003;9:1166–73.

[99] Mays E, Fontanges E, Fourcade N, et al. Bone loss after orthotopic liver transplantation. Am J Med 1994;97:445–50.

ELSEVIER
SAUNDERS

Clin Liver Dis 9 (2005) 183–189

CLINICS IN
LIVER DISEASE

Index

Note: Page numbers of article titles are in **boldface** type.

A

Absorption
  ethanol effects on, 74–76

Acetaldehyde
  as carcinogen, 157
  metabolism of, 14–16
  toxicity of, 14–16

Acid(s)
  amino
    alcohol effects on, 74–76
    for alcoholic hepatitis, 113–116
  folic
    alcohol effects on, 72
  omega 6 fatty
    alcohol effects on, 77

S-Adenosyl methionine
  for alcoholic liver disease, 143
  methionine and
    in alcohol metabolism, 16–17

S-Adenosyl-L-methione
  for alcoholic hepatitis, 120

ADH isozymes. See *Antidiuretic hormone (ADH) isozymes.*

Aflatoxin
  alcohol and, 155–156

African iron overload
  alcohol effects on, 93–94

Alcohol
  aflatoxin and, 155–156
  African iron overload effects of, 93–94
  carcinogens with
    effects of, 154–156
  β-carotene with
    toxic interactions of, 11–13
  diabetes mellitus and, 155
  effects on amino acids, 74–76
  effects on digestion, 76–78
  effects on HCV infection, **83–101.** See
    also *Hepatitis C virus (HCV)
    infection, alcohol effects on.*
  effects on minerals, 73–74

effects on vitamins, 67–73. See also
  Vitamin(s), alcohol effects on.
  HBV infection effects of, 90
  HCV infection and, **83–101,** 105–106,
    154–155
  hemochromatosis effects of, 91–93
  hepatocellular cancer effects of, 90–91
  immune surveillance and, 161–162
  in hepatocellular cancer, **151–169**
  liver disease associated with obesity
    effects of, 94–96
  metabolism of, **1–35**
    S-adenosyl methionine in, 16–17
    alcohol dehydrogenase pathway in,
      1–6
    antioxidants in, 18
    catalase pathway in, 13–14
    correction of alcohol-induced oxida-
      tive stress in liver in, 16–18
    dilinoleoyl-phosphadylcholine in,
      17–18
    extrahepatic, 18–22
    methionine in, 16–17
    microsomal ethanol oxidizing
      system in, 7–14
    nonoxidative, 22–23
    polyenyl-phosphatidylcholine in,
      17–18
    polymorphism of CYP2E1 and, 7–8
    vitamin E in, 18
  non–HFE-related iron overload
    syndromes effects of, 91–93
  oxidation of
    in stomach, 18–21
  oxidative stress in hepatocarcinogenesis
    and, 158
  retinoids and, 160–161
  retinol with
    toxic interactions of, 11–13
  smoking and, 154
  vinyl chloride and, 155–156

Alcohol dehydrogenase pathway
  ADH isozymes and, 1–6
  metabolic disorders and, 1–18
  microsomal ethanol oxidizing system
    and, 7–14

1089-3261/05/$ – see front matter © 2005 Elsevier Inc. All rights reserved.
doi:10.1016/S1089-3261(05)00009-7

Alcohol dehydrogenase polymorphism
  pathogenic role of, 6
Alcohol folate
  DNA methylation in hepatocellular
    cancer and, 159–160
Alcohol use
  in HCV infection history, 85–89
Alcoholic hepatitis. See also *Alcoholic
    liver disease.*
  inflammation in, 106–110
  pathogenesis of, 104–106
  prognosis for, 106
  treatment of, **103–134**
    S-adenosyl-L-methione in, 120
    anabolic steroids in, 118–119
    calcium channel blockers in, 121
    CAM in, 121–122
    case reports in, 122
    colchicine in, 119–120
    corticosteroids in, 111–113
    future directions in, 124–125
    hepatic regeneration promoters in,
      116–107
    new agents in, 123–124
    pentoxifylline in, 123–124
    polyunsaturated lecithin in, 121
    propylthiouracil, 117–118
    supplemental amino acids in,
      113–116
Alcoholic liver disease. See also
    Alcoholic hepatitis.
  antigenic adduct formation in, 64
  chemokines in, 62
  conditions associated with, 48–49
  cytotoxicity of, 59
  differential diagnosis of
    pathologic, 49–51
  fibrogenesis in, 59
  HCV infection in, 105–106
  hyaline bodies in, 60–62
  IL-6 in, 63
  IL-8 in, 63–64
  immune complexes in, 59–60
  immunology of, **55–66**
  Kupffer cells in, 56–57
  liver transplantation for, 145, **171–181**
    allograft cellular rejection after, 175
    candidate selection for, 172–173
    compliance after, 176
    described, 173–175
    osteopenia after, 177
    posttransplant issues, 174
      social issues, 175–176
    pretransplant issues
      social issues, 171–172
    quality of life after, 176
    recidivism after, 175–176
    recurrent disease after, 174–175

  survival rates, 174
  tumors after, 176–177
lymphocytes in, 57–59
morphology of, **37–53**
neutrophils in, 57
nutritional aspects of, **67–81**
pathogenesis of, 104–106
prevention of, 144–145
recurrence of
  after liver transplantation, 174–175
steatohepatitis in, 41–45
  grading of, 48
  progression to cirrhosis, 45–48
  staging of, 48
steatosis in, 37–41
treatment of
  complications of
    ascites, 138
    endocrine function disorders,
      139–140
    esophageal varices, 137
    hematologic effects of, 138
    hepatic encephalopathy,
      140–141
    hepatic osteodystrophy, 139
    hepatorenal syndrome,
      138–139
    HPS, 139
    long-term, 137–141
    PPHTN, 139
  drug toxicity with, 144
  long-term, **135–149**
    S-adenosyl methione in, 143
    anabolic steroids in, 141–142
    colchicine in, 142
    pharmacologic therapy in,
      141–143
    propylthiouracil in, 142
    silymarin in, 142–143
    ursodeoxycholic acid in, 141
  nutrition in, 143
  overview of, 136–137
  surgery in
    risk factors in, 144
  tumor necrosis factor-α in, 62–63
Alcohol-induced hepatocellular cancer, 90–91,
  151–169
  mechanisms of, 156–162
Alcoholism
  effects on vitamins, 67–73
Allograft cellular rejection
  after liver transplantation, 175
Amino acids
  alcohol effects on, 74–76
  for alcoholic hepatitis, 113–116
Anabolic steroids
  for alcoholic hepatitis, 118–119
  for alcoholic liver disease, 141–142

Antidiuretic hormone (ADH) isozymes
  alcohol dehydrogenase pathway and,
    1–6
Antioxidant(s)
  in alcohol metabolism, 18
Arginine
  alcohol effects on, 74
Ascites
  alcoholic liver disease and
    management of, 138

C

Caffeine
  alcohol effects on, 77–78
Calcium
  alcohol effects on, 73
Calcium channel blockers
  for alcoholic hepatitis, 121
Cancer
  hepatocellular
    alcohol in. See also *Hepatocellular
      cancer, alcohol-induced.*
    alcohol-induced, 90–91, **151–169**
Carcinogen(s)
  acetaldehyde as, 157
  alcohol with
    effects of, 154–156
Carnitine
  alcohol effects on, 76
β-Carotene
  alcohol effects on, 76
  alcohol with
    toxic interactions of, 11–13
Catalase pathway
  in alcohol metabolism, 13–14
Chemokine(s)
  in alcoholic liver disease, 62
Choline
  alcohol effects on, 76
Ciancobalamine
  alcohol effects on, 71
Cirrhosis
  alcoholic
    immunity in, 143
    nutrition in, 143
    steatohepatitis progression to
      in alcoholic liver disease, 45–48
Colchicine
  for alcoholic hepatitis, 119–120
  for alcoholic liver disease, 142

Complementary and alternative
    medicines (CAM)
  for alcoholic hepatitis, 121–122
Compliance
  after liver transplantation, 176
Copper
  alcohol effects on, 73
Corticosteroid(s)
  for alcoholic hepatitis, 111–113
CYP2E1
  in alcohol metabolism
    nutritional role of, 9
  in extrahepatic tissues, 21–22
  in Kupffer cells, 21–22
  in nonalcoholic steatohepatitis, 21–22
  physiologic role of, 22
  polymorphism of
    in alcohol metabolism, 7–8
Cytochrome P450 2EI
  alcohol in hepatocellular cancer and,
    157–158
Cytotoxicity
  in alcoholic liver disease, 59

D

Diabetes mellitus
  alcohol and, 155
Digestion
  alcohol effects on, 76–78
Dilinoleoyl-phosphadylcholine
  in alcohol metabolism, 17–18
Drug(s)
  for alcoholic liver disease, 141–143
Drug toxicity
  in alcoholic cirrhotics, 144

E

Encephalopathy(ies)
  hepatic
    alcoholic liver disease and
      management of, 140–141
Endocrine function disorders
  alcoholic liver disease and
    management of, 139–140
Esophageal varices
  alcoholic liver disease and
    management of, 137
Ethanol
  absorption effects of, 74–76
  amino acid effects of, 74–76

digestion effects of, 76–78
  minerals effects of, 73–74
  vitamins effects of, 67–73. See also
    Vitamin(s), alcohol effects on.

Extrahepatic alcohol metabolism, 18–22

Extrahepatic tissues
  CYP2E1 in, 21–22

F

Fibrogenesis
  in alcoholic liver disease, 59

Folic acid
  alcohol effects on, 72

G

L-Glutamine
  alcohol effects on, 75

Glutathione
  alcohol effects on, 77

Glycine
  alcohol effects on, 75

H

HBV infection. See *Hepatitis B virus
  (HBV) infection.*

HCV infection. See *Hepatitis C virus
  (HCV) infection.*

Hemochromatosis
  alcohol effects on, 91–93

Hepatic encephalopathy
  alcoholic liver disease and
    management of, 140–141

Hepatic osteodystrophy
  alcoholic liver disease and
    management of, 139

Hepatic steatosis, 5–6

Hepatitis
  alcoholic
    treatment of, **103–134.** See also
      *Alcoholic hepatitis,
      treatment of.*
  viral
    HIV coinfected with
      alcohol effects on, 91
    surveillance of
      recommendations for
        in alcoholic liver
          disease, 144–145

Hepatitis B virus (HBV) infection
  alcohol and, 154–155
  alcohol effects on, 90

Hepatitis C virus (HCV) infection
  alcohol and, 154–155
  alcohol effects on, **83–101**
    studies of, 84–85
      treatment-related, 89–90
  in alcoholic(s)
    prevalence of, 84
  in alcoholic liver disease, 105–106
  natural history of
    alcohol use in, 85–89
  prevalence of, 84
  treatment of
    alcohol effects on, 89–90

Hepatocarcinogenesis
  oxidative stress in
    alcohol and, 158

Hepatocellular cancer
  alcohol-induced, 90–91, **151–169**
    epidemiology of, 152–154
    mechanisms of, 156–162
  DNA methylation in
    alcohol folate, B_6, B_{12} and,
      159–160
  in alcoholic liver disease prevention, 144
  prevalence of, 151

Hepatopulmonary syndrome (HPS)
  alcoholic liver disease and
    management of, 139

Hepatorenal syndrome
  alcoholic liver disease and
    management of, 138–139

Homocysteine
  alcohol effects on, 77

HPS. See *Hepatopulmonary syndrome (HPS).*

Human immunodeficiency virus
  (HIV) infection
  viral hepatitis coinfected with
    alcohol effects on, 91

Hyaline bodies
  in alcoholic liver disease, 60–62

I

IL. See *Interleukin(s) (IL).*

Immune complexes
  in alcoholic liver disease, 59–60

Immune surveillance
  alcohol and, 161–162

Immunity
  in alcoholic liver disease, 143

Immunology
    of alcoholic liver disease, **55–66**
Interleukin(s) (IL)
    IL-6
        in alcoholic liver disease, 63
    IL-8
        in alcoholic liver disease, 63–64
Iron
    alcohol effects on, 73
Isozyme(s)
    ADH
        alcohol dehydrogenase pathway
            and, 1–6

K

Kupffer cells
    CYP2E1 in, 21–22
    in alcoholic liver disease, 56–57

L

Lecithin
    polyunsaturated
        for alcoholic hepatitis, 121
Lecithin (phosphatidyl choline)
    alcohol effects on, 77
Lithium
    alcohol effects on, 74
Liver
    regeneration of
        promoters of
            in alcoholic hepatitis,
                116–117
Liver disease
    alcoholic. See *Alcoholic liver disease.*
    obesity-related
        alcohol effects on, 94–96
Liver macrophages, 56–57
Liver transplantation
    for alcoholic liver disease, 145,
        171–181. See also *Alcoholic liver
        disease, liver transplantation for.*
Lymphocyte(s)
    in alcoholic liver disease, 57–59

M

Macrophage(s)
    liver, 56–57
Magnesium
    alcohol effects on, 73–74

Metabolism
    of alcohol, **1–35.** See also *Alcohol,
        metabolism of.*
Methionine
    S-adenosyl methionine
        in alcohol metabolism, 16–17
    alcohol effects on, 75
Microsomal ethanol oxidizing system
    alcohol dehydrogenase pathway and,
        7–14
Mineral(s)
    alcohol effects on, 73–74

N

NAFLD. See *Nonalcoholic fatty liver
    disease (NAFLD).*
Neutrophil(s)
    in alcoholic liver disease, 57
Niacin
    alcohol effects on, 71
Nonalcoholic fatty liver disease (NAFLD)
    obesity and, 94
Nonalcoholic steatohepatitis
    CYP2E1 in, 21–22
Non–HFE-related iron overload syndromes
    alcohol effects on, 91–93
Nutrition
    in alcoholic liver disease, 143
Nutritional status
    in alcoholic liver disease, **67–81**

O

Obesity
    liver disease associated with
        alcohol effects on, 94–96
Omega 6 fatty acids
    alcohol effects on, 77
Osteodystrophy
    hepatic
        alcoholic liver disease and
            management of, 139
Osteopenia
    after liver transplantation, 177
Oxidative stress
    alcohol-induced
        in liver
            correction of, 16–18
        in hepatocarcinogenesis
            alcohol and, 158

P

Panthetine
    alcohol effects on, 77
Pentoxifylline
    for alcoholic hepatitis, 123–124
Phosphatidyl choline
    alcohol effects on, 77
Phosphorus
    alcohol effects on, 74
Polyenyl-phosphatidylcholine
    in alcohol metabolism, 17–18
Polyunsaturated lecithin
    for alcoholic hepatitis, 121
Portopulmonary hypertension (PPHTN)
    alcoholic liver disease and
        management of, 139
Potassium
    alcohol effects on, 74
PPHTN. See *Portopulmonary
    hypertension (PPHTN).*
Propylthiouracil
    for alcoholic hepatitis, 117–118
    for alcoholic liver disease, 142
Pyridoxine
    alcohol effects on, 71

Q

Quality of life
    after liver transplantation, 176

R

Recidivism
    after liver transplantation, 175–176
Retinoid(s)
    alcohol and, 160–161
Retinol
    alcohol effects on, 67–70
    alcohol with
        toxic interactions of, 11–13
Riboflavin
    alcohol effects on, 71

S

Selenium
    alcohol effects on, 74
Serine
    alcohol effects on, 75

Silymarin
    for alcoholic liver disease, 142–143
Smoking
    alcohol and, 154
Steatohepatitis
    in alcoholic liver disease, 41–45
    nonalcoholic
        CYP2E1 in, 21–22
    to cirrhosis
        progression of
            in alcoholic liver disease,
                45–48
Steatosis
    hepatic, 5–6
    in alcoholic liver disease, 37–41
Steroid(s)
    anabolic
        for alcoholic hepatitis, 118–119
        for alcoholic liver disease, 141–142
Stomach
    oxidation of alcohol in, 18–21
Stress
    oxidative
        alcohol-induced
            in liver
                correction of, 16–18
        in hepatocarcinogenesis
            alcohol and, 158

T

Taurine
    alcohol effects on, 76
Thiamine
    alcohol effects on, 70–71
Transplantation
    liver. See *Liver transplantation.*
Tryptophan
    alcohol effects on, 76
Tumor(s)
    after liver transplantation, 176–177
Tumor necrosis factor-α
    in alcoholic liver disease, 62–63

U

Ursodeoxycholic acid
    for alcoholic liver disease, 141

V

Varice(es)
    esophageal
        alcoholic liver disease and
            management of, 137

Vinyl chloride
    alcohol and, 155–156
Viral hepatitis
    HIV coinfected with
        alcohol effects on, 91
    surveillance of
        recommendations for
            in alcoholic liver disease
                prevention, 144–145
Vitamin(s)
    alcohol effects on, 67–73
        A (retinol), 67–70
        B complex, 70
        B_1 (thiamine), 70–71
        B_2 (riboflavin), 71
        B_3 (niacin), 71
        B_6 (pyridoxine), 71
        B_{12} (ciancobalamine), 71
        C, 72
        D, 72
        E, 73
        folic acid, 72
        K, 73
    B_6
        DNA methylation in hepatocellular
            cancer and, 159–160
    B_{12}
        DNA methylation in hepatocellular
            cancer and, 159–160
    E
        in alcohol metabolism, 18

Z

Zinc
    alcohol effects on, 74

Changing Your Address?

Make sure your subscription changes too! When you notify us of your new address, you can help make our job easier by including an exact copy of your Clinics label number with your old address (see illustration below.) This number identifies you to our computer system and will speed the processing of your address change. Please be sure this label number accompanies your old address and your corrected address—you can send an old Clinics label with your number on it or just copy it exactly and send it to the address listed below.

We appreciate your help in our attempt to give you continuous coverage. Thank you.

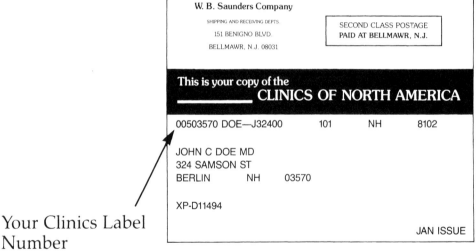

W. B. Saunders Company

SHIPPING AND RECEIVING DEPTS.
151 BENIGNO BLVD.
BELLMAWR, N.J. 08031

SECOND CLASS POSTAGE
PAID AT BELLMAWR, N.J.

This is your copy of the
_____ CLINICS OF NORTH AMERICA

00503570 DOE—J32400   101   NH   8102

JOHN C DOE MD
324 SAMSON ST
BERLIN   NH   03570

XP-D11494

JAN ISSUE

Your Clinics Label Number
Copy it exactly or send your label along with your address to:
W.B. Saunders Company, Customer Service
Orlando, FL 32887-4800
Call Toll Free 1-800-654-2452

Please allow four to six weeks for delivery of new subscriptions and for processing address changes.

Order your subscription today. Simply complete and detach this card and drop it in the mail to receive the best clinical information in your field.

❑ **Adolescent Medicine Clinics**
❑ Individual $95
❑ Institutions $133
❑ *In-training $48

❑ **Anesthesiology**
❑ Individual $175
❑ Institutions $270
❑ *In-training $88

❑ **Cardiology**
❑ Individual $170
❑ Institutions $266
❑ *In-training $85

❑ **Chest Medicine**
❑ Individual $185
❑ Institutions $285

❑ **Child and Adolescent Psychiatry**
❑ Individual $175
❑ Institutions $265
❑ *In-training $88

❑ **Critical Care**
❑ Individual $165
❑ Institutions $266
❑ *In-training $83

❑ **Dental**
❑ Individual $150
❑ Institutions $242

❑ **Emergency Medicine**
❑ Individual $170
❑ Institutions $263
❑ *In-training $85
❑ Send CME info

❑ **Facial Plastic Surgery**
❑ Individual $199
❑ Institutions $300

❑ **Foot and Ankle**
Individual $160
Institutions $232

❑ **Gastroenterology**
❑ Individual $190
❑ Institutions $276

❑ **Gastrointestinal Endoscopy**
❑ Individual $190
❑ Institutions $276

❑ **Hand**
❑ Individual $205
❑ Institutions $319

❑ **Heart Failure (NEW in 2005!)**
❑ Individual $99
❑ Institutions $149
❑ *In-training $49

❑ **Hematology/ Oncology**
❑ Individual $210
❑ Institutions $315

❑ **Immunology & Allergy**
❑ Individual $165
❑ Institutions $266

❑ **Infectious Disease**
❑ Individual $165
❑ Institutions $272

❑ **Clinics in Liver Disease**
❑ Individual $165
❑ Institutions $234

❑ **Medical**
❑ Individual $140
❑ Institutions $244
❑ *In-training $70
❑ Send CME info

❑ **MRI**
❑ Individual $190
❑ Institutions $290
❑ *In-training $95
❑ Send CME info

❑ **Neuroimaging**
❑ Individual $190
❑ Institutions $290
❑ *In-training $95
❑ Send CME inf0

❑ **Neurologic**
❑ Individual $175
❑ Institutions $275

❑ **Obstetrics & Gynecology**
❑ Individual $175
❑ Institutions $288

❑ **Occupational and Environmental Medicine**
❑ Individual $120
❑ Institutions $166
❑ *In-training $60

❑ **Ophthalmology**
❑ Individual $190
❑ Institutions $325

❑ **Oral & Maxillofacial Surgery**
❑ Individual $180
❑ Institutions $280
❑ *In-training $90

❑ **Orthopedic**
❑ Individual $180
❑ Institutions $295
❑ *In-training $90

❑ **Otolaryngologic**
❑ Individual $199
❑ Institutions $350

❑ **Pediatric**
❑ Individual $135
❑ Institutions $246
❑ *In-training $68
❑ Send CME info

❑ **Perinatology**
❑ Individual $155
❑ Institutions $237
❑ *In-training $78
❑ Send CME inf0

❑ **Plastic Surgery**
❑ Individual $245
❑ Institutions $370

❑ **Podiatric Medicine & Surgery**
❑ Individual $170
❑ Institutions $266

❑ **Primary Care**
❑ Individual $135
❑ Institutions $223

❑ **Psychiatric**
❑ Individual $170
❑ Institutions $288

❑ **Radiologic**
❑ Individual $220
❑ Institutions $331
❑ *In-training $110
❑ Send CME info

❑ **Sports Medicine**
❑ Individual $180
❑ Institutions $277

❑ **Surgical**
❑ Individual $190
❑ Institutions $299
❑ *In-training $95

❑ **Thoracic Surgery (formerly Chest Surgery)**
❑ Individual $175
❑ Institutions $255
❑ *In-training $88

❑ **Urologic**
❑ Individual $195
❑ Institutions $307
❑ *In-training $98
❑ Send CME info

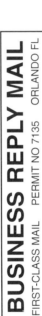

BUSINESS REPLY MAIL

FIRST-CLASS MAIL   PERMIT NO 7135   ORLANDO FL

POSTAGE WILL BE PAID BY ADDRESSEE

PERIODICALS ORDER FULFILLMENT DEPT
ELSEVIER
6277 SEA HARBOR DR
ORLANDO FL 32821-9816